Fundamentals of Renal Pathology

Fundamentals of Renal Pathology

Agnes B. Fogo
Editor

Jan Bruijn
Arthur H. Cohen
Robert B. Colvin
J. Charles Jennette
Coeditors

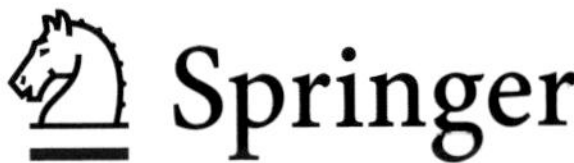

Agnes B. Fogo, M.D.
Vanderbilt University Medical Center
Nashville, TN, USA

Arthur H. Cohen, M.D.
Cedars-Sinai Medical Center
UCLA School of Medicine
Los Angeles, CA, USA

J. Charles Jennette, M.D.
University of North Carolina
Chapel Hill, NC, USA

Jan A. Bruijn, M.D., Ph.D.
Leiden University Medical Center
Leiden, the Netherlands

Robert B. Colvin, M.D.
Massachusetts General Hospital
Boston, MA, USA

Library of Congress Control Number: 2005939064

ISBN-10: 0-387-31126-2 e-ISBN 0-387-31127-0
ISBN-13: 978-0-387-31126-5

Printed on acid-free paper.

Printed in the United States of America.

9 8 7 6 5 4 3 2 (corrected printing, 2008)

springer.com

Table of Contents

Section I
Renal Anatomy and Basic Concepts and Methods in Renal Pathology

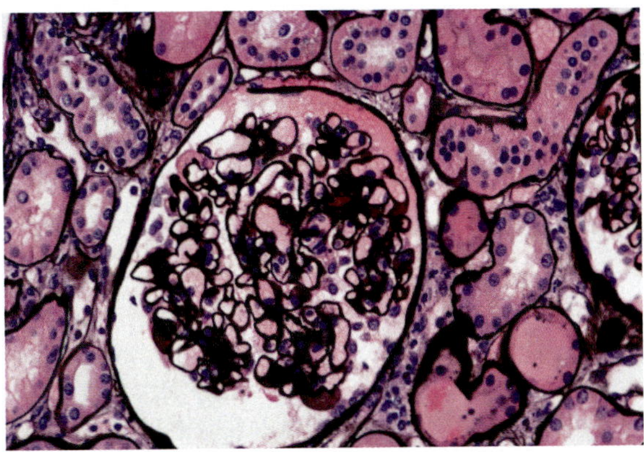

FIGURE 1.3. Normal glomerulus with surrounding normal tubules and interstitium (Jones silver stain).

system. Cortical parenchyma extends into spaces between adjacent pyramids; this portion of the cortex is known as the columns of Bertin. A medullary pyramid with surrounding cortical parenchyma, which includes both columns of Bertin as well as the subcapsular cortex, constitutes a renal lobe. The collecting system consists of the pelvis, which represents the expanded upper portion of the ureter, and is more or less funnel shaped. Each pelvis has two or three major branches known as the major calyces. Each calyx divides further into three or four smaller branches known as minor calyces, each usually receiving one medullary papilla.

Each kidney contains approximately 1 million nephrons, each composed of a glomerulus and attached tubules. Glomeruli are spherical collections of interconnected capillaries within a space (Bowman's space) lined by flattened parietal epithelial cells (Fig. 1.3). Bowman's space is continuous with the tubules, with the orifice of the proximal tubule generally at the pole opposite the glomerular hilus, where the afferent and efferent arterioles enter and leave, respectively. The outer aspects of the glomerular capillaries are covered by a layer of visceral epithelial cells or podocytes. Each visceral epithelial cell has a large body containing the nucleus and cytoplasmic extensions, which divide, forming small finger-like processes that interdigitate with similar structures from adjacent cells and cover the capillaries. These interdigitating processes, known as pedicles, are also called foot processes because of their appearance on transmission electron microscopy. The space between adjacent foot processes is known as the filtration slit; adjacent foot processes are joined together by a thin membrane known as the slit-pore diaphragm. Epithelial cells cover the glomerular capillary basement membrane, a three-layer structure with a central thick layer slightly electron dense (lamina densa) and thinner electron lucent layers beneath epithelial and endothelial cells (lamina rara externa and lamina rara interna, respectively) (Fig. 1.4). The glomerular basement membrane is composed predominately of type IV collagen with small amount type V collagen, laminin, and proteoglycans, predominantly heparan sulfate. In addition, entactin and fibronectin are present. The glomerular basement membrane in adults measures approximately 340 to 360 nanometers (nm) in thickness and is significantly thicker in men than in women. The endothelial cells are thin and have multiple fenestrae, each measuring approximately 80 nm in diameter. The capillary tufts are supported by the mesangium, which represents the intraglomerular continuation of the arteriolar walls. The mesangium has two components. The extracellular one, *mesangial matrix*, has many structural, compositional, and, therefore, tinctorial properties similar to basement membrane. The cells of the mesangium are known as *mesangial cells*, of which there are two types: modified smooth muscle cells, representing greater than 95% of the cellular population, and bone marrow–derived cells, representing the remainder. Mesangial cells have numerous functions including contraction, production of extracellular matrix, secretion of inflammatory and other active mediators, phagocytosis, and migration from the central zone where they are normally situated (Fig. 1.5).

The proteoglycans of the glomerular basement membrane are negatively charged; similarly, the surface of both epithelial and endothelial cells are anionically charged because of sialoglycoproteins in the cellular coats. Both of these negatively charged structures are responsible for the *charge-selective barrier* to filtration of capillary contents. The basement membrane, which, along with the fenestrated endothelial cell, allows for ready filtration of water and small substances, is known as the *size-selective*

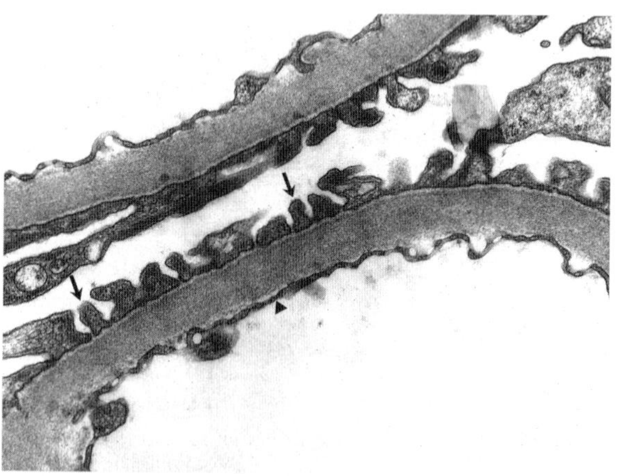

FIGURE 1.4. Portion of glomerular capillary wall by electron microscopy. Individual foot processes of visceral epithelial cells (arrows) cover the basement membrane and endothelial cell cytoplasm (arrowhead) lines the lumen.

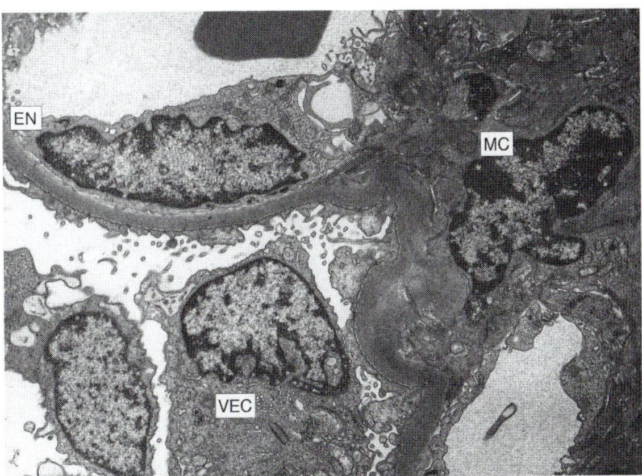

FIGURE 1.5. Portion of glomerulus indicating different cell types: capillary endothelial cell (EN), visceral epithelial cell (VEC), and mesangial cell (MC) (electron microscopy).

barrier. The visceral epithelial cell in the adult is responsible for the production and maintenance of basement membrane.

The remaining portion of the nephron is divided into *proximal tubules*, which are often convoluted, the *loop of Henle*, with both descending and ascending limbs, and the *distal tubule*. The proximal tubular cells have well-developed closely packed microvillous luminal surfaces known as the brush border. The cells are larger than those of the distal tubules, which have relatively few surface microvilli. Each tubule is surrounded completely by a basement membrane. Adjacent tubular basement membranes are in almost direct contact with one another and separated by a small amount of connective tissue known as the interstitium, which contain peritubular capillaries (Fig. 1.6). At the vascular pole of the glomerulus and

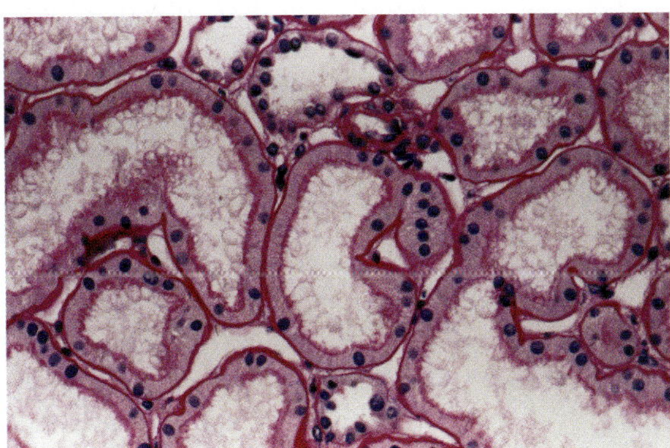

FIGURE 1.6. Normal cortical tubules, interstitium, and peritubular capillaries; most of the tubules are proximal, with well-defined brush borders (PAS stain).

the site of entrance of the afferent arteriole, the cells of the arteriolar wall are modified into secretory cells known as juxtaglomerular cells; these produce and secrete renin, contained in granules. The macula densa, a portion of the distal tubule at the glomerular hilus, is characterized by smaller and more crowded distal tubular cells, which are in contact with the juxtaglomerular cells. Surrounding the macula densa and afferent arteriole are lacis cells, which are mesenchymal cells similar to mesangial cells.

Examination of Renal Tissue

Because of the types of diseases and the renal components that are abnormal, the preparation of tissue specimens for examination is somewhat complex considering the required methods of study. These include sophisticated *light microscopy*, immunofluorescence, and electron microscopy. For light microscopy, the elucidation of lesions of glomeruli mandates that a variety of histochemical stains be used and that tissue sections be cut thinner than for other tissues. Furthermore, to take best advantage of the stains, many investigators and renal pathologists have found that formalin, Zenker's solution, or many of the more commonly used fixatives result in substandard preparations. Consequently, alcoholic Bouin's solution (Duboseq-Brasil) is the fixative of choice. For the elucidation of glomerular structure and pathology, it is necessary that the extracellular matrix components (basement membrane, mesangial matrix) be preferentially stained. Table 1.1 indicates staining characteristic of normal and abnormal renal structures. In paraffin-embedded sections, the hematoxylin and eosin stain does not ordinarily allow for distinction of extracellular matrix from cytoplasm in a clear or convincing manner. Periodic acid-Schiff (PAS), periodic acid-methenamine silver (Jones), and Masson's trichrome stains all provide excellent definition of extracellular material. Each stain has its advantages and disadvantages, and as a rule, all are used in evaluating renal tissues especially biopsies. The PAS reagent stains glomerular basement membranes, mesangial matrix, and tubular basement membranes red (positive), while the Jones stain colors the same components black, providing clear contrast between positively and negatively staining structures. Masson's trichrome stain colors extracellular glomerular matrix and tubular basement membranes blue, clearly distinguished from cells and abnormal material that accumulates in pathologic circumstances. Congo red, elastic tissue, and other stains are employed when indicated. The tissue sections should be no greater than 2 to 3μm in thickness, for the definition of glomerular pathology, especially regarding cellularity, is dependent on sections of this thickness. The ability to detect subtle pathologic abnormalities is enhanced with thinner sections. Especially for glomerular diseases, *immunohistochemistry* is necessary for evaluation renal tissues, especially for diagnosing glomerular diseases. Most laboratories utilize *immunofluorescence* for identifying and localizing immunoglobulins, complement, fibrin, and other

TABLE 1.1. Staining characteristics of selected normal and abnormal renal structures

	Stain		
	PAS	Jones	Masson's trichrome
Basement membrane	Red	Black	Deep blue
Mesangial matrix	Red	Black	Deep blue
Interstitial collagen	Negative	Negative	Pale blue
Cell cytoplasm (normal)	Negative (most)	Negative	Rust/orange-granular
Immune complex deposits	Negative to slightly positive	Negative	Bright red-orange homogeneous
"Insudative lesions"	Negative to slightly positive	Negative	Bright red-orange homogeneous
Fibrin	Slightly positive	Negative	Bright red-orange fibrillar
Other			
Plasma protein precipitates (intra- or extracellular)	Slightly positive	Negative	Bright red-orange homogeneous
Amyloid (Congo Red positive)	Negative	Negative (sometimes positive)	Light blue-orange
Tubular casts (Tamm-Horsfall protein)	Red	Gray to black	Light blue

PAS, periodic acid-Schiff.

immune substances within renal tissues; fluorescein-labeled antibodies to the following are used: immunoglobulin G (IgG), IgA, IgM, C1q, C3, albumin, fibrin, and kappa and lambda immunoglobulin light chains. For transplant biopsies, anitbody to C4d is routinely utilized. Fluorescence positivity in glomeruli is described as *granular* or *linear* (Fig. 1.7). Regard-

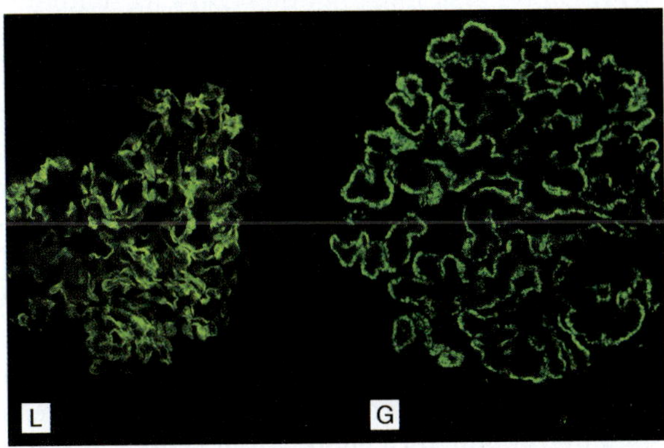

FIGURE 1.7. Glomerular immunofluorescence indicating linear (L) and granular (G) capillary wall staining for immunoglobulin G (IgG).

TABLE 1.2. Immune deposits

IF	LM	EM
Granular	Trichrome stain bright red-orange	Electron dense
Linear	Not visible	Not visible

EM, electron microscopy; IF, immunofluorescence; LM, light microscopy.

less of the immunopathologic mechanisms responsible for the granular deposits, there is an electron microscopic counterpart to granular deposits; by electron microscopy, extracellular masses of electron-dense material correspond to the deposits. The granular deposits can be appreciated in tissue prepared for light microscopy; this is best demonstrated and documented with the use of Masson's trichrome stain, where granular deposits appear as bright fuchsinophilic (orange, red-orange) smooth homogeneous structures. There is no regular ultrastructural or light microscopic counterpart to linear staining (Table 1.2). *Electron microscopy* is routinely utilized in the study of renal tissues. For glomerular and some tubulo-interstitial diseases this method is mandatory and helps localize deposits, detects extremely small deposits, and documents alterations of cellular and basement membrane structure. Immunofluorescence and electron microscopy are also often necessary and helpful in diagnosing other tubular, interstitial, and vascular lesions.

The typical appearances and tinctorial properties with routinely used stains of normal and abnormal renal structures are provided in Table 1.1.

Tamm-Horsfall Protein (THP) (Also Known as Uromodulin)

Tamm-Horsfall protein is a large glycoprotein (mucoprotein) produced only by cells of the thick ascending limb of the loop of Henle. While it has many physiologic functions, for the pathologist interested in renal tissue changes it provides important information regarding tubular structure and integrity. This glycoprotein, when precipitated in gel form in distal tubules, forms a cast of the tubular lumen, which may be passed in the urine as a hyaline cast. Thus, Tamm-Horsfall protein is the fundamental constituent of urinary casts. In tissue sections, the casts are strongly PAS positive and can easily be recognized. The structural value of this feature is that the cast material, in a variety of pathologic states, may be found in abnormal locations and therefore may provide evidence regarding pathogenesis of certain diseases and their pathophysiologic consequences. Tamm-Horsfall protein has been identified primarily in three major abnormal sites: (1) the proximal nephron, (2) the renal interstitium and occasionally intrarenal capillaries and veins, and (3) in perihilar locations. It has been documented that with intra- or extrarenal obstruction and/or reflux, THP may be found in proximal tubules and in glomerular urinary spaces, the result of retrograde flow in the nephron. Escape of THP from within the nephron into the interstitium and peritubular capillaries has been documented to occur with tubular wall disruption. There are four major mechanisms proposed for this finding: (1) increased intranephron pressure (reflux, obstruction), which can cause rupture of the tubular wall and spillage of contents locally; (2) destruction of tubular walls by infiltrating leukocytes (as in any acute interstitial nephritis); collagenases produced by infiltrating cells, especially monocytes, can dissolve basement membranes and concomitant epithelial cell damage can result in tubular wall defects; (3) in acute tubular necrosis (especially of ischemic type) both cell death and basement membrane loss have been described; interstitial and capillary and venous THP is uncommonly observed; and (4) intrinsic defects of tubular basement membranes (as in juvenile nephronophthisis), which likely result in loss of compliance of tubular walls and, in addition to cyst formation, may also lead to dissolution of part of the walls with escape of luminal contents. In all of the above, it is clear that while other tubular contents may also be in abnormal locations, it is Tamm-Horsfall protein that has the morphologic and tinctorial features that allow microscopists to identify it and use it as a marker of urine. Tamm-Horsfall protein is a weak immunogen; initially it was thought that its escape from tubules was, in large part, immunologically responsible for progression of chronic tubulo-interstitial damage in the disorders characterized by this feature. However, despite the presence of serum anti-THP antibodies in patients with reflux nephropathy, the pathogenic role of THP in immunologic renal injury is uncertain and probably not very important. Tamm-Horsfall protein has been documented to bind and inactivate interleukin-1 (IL-1) and tumor necrosis factor (TNF).

General Pathology of Renal Structures

Before embarking on a consideration of various renal diseases, a discussion of basic abnormalities that characterize the renal structures is presented first.

Glomeruli

Increased cellularity (hypercellularity) may result from increase in intrinsic cells (mesangial, visceral epithelial or endothelial cells) or from accumulation of leukocytes in capillary lumina, beneath endothelial cells, or in the mesangium. Although not entirely correct, glomerular lesions with increased cells in the tufts are often known as proliferative glomerulonephritis. Accumulation of cells and fibrin within the urinary space is known as a crescent (see below).

Increase in extracellular matrix implies an increase in mesangial matrix or basement membrane material. In the former instance, this may be in a uniform and diffuse pattern in all lobules or cause a nodular appearance to the mesangium. Increased basement membrane material takes the form of thickened basement membranes, an abnormality that is best appreciated by electron microscopy.

Sclerosis refers to increased extracellular matrix and other material leading to obliteration of capillaries and solidification of all or part of the tufts. Sclerosis (glomerular scarring) may be associated with obliteration of the urinary space by collagen along with increased extracellular matrix in the capillary tufts. When the entire glomerulus is involved, this is known as complete sclerosis; an older and less precise term is *glomerular hyalinization*. Segmental glomerulosclerosis implies a completely different pathologic process and often a disease. With segmental sclerosis, only portions of the capillary tufts are involved; capillaries are obliterated by increased extracellular matrix and/or large precipitates of plasma protein known as insudates.

Crescents represent accumulation of cells and extracellular material in the urinary space. Crescents are the result of severe capillary wall damage with disruptions in continuity and spillage of fibrin from inside the damaged capillaries into the urinary spaces. This is associated with proliferation of visceral and perhaps parietal epithelial cells and accumulation of monocytes and other blood cells in the urinary space. The cellular composition of the crescent varies depending on the type of disease and associated damage to the basement membrane of Bowman's capsule. Crescents most commonly heal by organization (scar formation). With an admixture of cells and collagen, the crescent is considered fibrocellular, and with only collagen in the urinary space, the crescent is designated as fibrotic.

Peripheral migration and interposition of mesangium: Mesangial cells and often matrix extend from the central lobular portion of the tuft into the peripheral capillary wall, migrating between endothelial cell and basement membrane and causing capillary wall thickening with two layers of extracellular matrix. This two-layer or double-contour appearance may involve a few or all capillaries.

Alteration in visceral epithelial cell morphology: This abnormality requires the electron microscope to detect. In association with protein loss across the glomerular capillary wall, the epithelial cells change shape; the foot processes retract and swell, resulting in loss of individual foot processes and a near solid mass of cytoplasm covering the glomerular basement membrane. This loss or *effacement of foot processes* is also incorrectly known as fusion because it was initially thought adjacent foot processes fused with one another.

Tubules

Tubular cells may exhibit a variety of degenerative changes, or may undergo acute reversible and irreversible damage (necrosis). The degenerative lesions are often in the form of intracellular accumulations, manifestations of either local metabolic abnormalities or systemic processes. For example, lipid inclusions in proximal and, less commonly, distal tubular cells result from hyperlipidemia and lipiduria of nephrotic syndrome, and protein reabsorption droplets ("hyaline droplets") accumulate in proximal tubular cells in association with albuminuria and its reabsorption by tubular epithelium. Additional locally induced abnormalities include uniform fine cytoplasmic vacuolization consequent to hypertonic solution infusion (e.g., mannitol, sucrose). Tubular cells may be sites of "storage" of hemosiderin in patients with chronic intravascular hemolysis, high iron load, or glomerular hematuria. Few metabolic storage diseases affect tubular epithelium; among others are cystinosis with crystals and glycogen storage diseases and diabetes mellitus with abundant intracellular glycogen. Vacuoles, especially large and irregular, may be associated with hypokalemia.

On the other hand, reversible and irreversible changes are features of acute tubular necrosis. These include loss of brush border staining for proximal cells, diffuse flattening of cells with resulting dilatation of lumina, loss of individual lining cells, and sloughing of cells into lumina. Manifestations of repair or regeneration include cytoplasmic basophilia and mitotic figures.

The morphologic features of atrophy of tubules include not only diminution in caliber, but more importantly irregular thickening and wrinkling of basement membranes. Adjacent tubules are invariably separated from one another in this circumstance. The intervening interstitium is almost always fibrotic, with or without accompanying inflammation. Other structural forms of tubular atrophy include uniform flattening of cells, hyaline casts in dilated lumina, and close approximation of tubules, resulting in a thyroid-like appearance to the parenchyma.

Interstitium

There are limited structural manifestations of interstitial injury. Commonly observed are edema, inflammation, and fibrosis. Both cortical edema and fibrosis are associated with separation of normally closely apposed tubules. With edema only, the tubular basement membranes are of normal thickness and contour. In contrast, with fibrosis the tubules are invariably atrophied with thickened and irregularly contoured basement membranes. The distinction between an acute and a chronic interstitial process is made based on the presence of edema (acute) or fibrosis (chronic) regardless of the character of any infiltrating leukocytes. With interstitial inflammation, especially when acute, the leukocytes, which gain access to the interstitium from the peritubular capillaries, usually extend into the walls of tubules. During this process, there may be damage to and destruction of tubular basement membranes as well as degeneration of epithelial cells. This often results in spillage of tubular contents into the interstitium.

The type(s) of cells in an interstitial inflammatory infiltrate depend(s) on the nature of the inflammatory process. For example, polymorphonuclear leukocytes, *as expected*, are present in early phases of many bacterial infections; however, they do not remain and are usually replaced by lymphocytes, plasma cells, and monocytes approximately 7 to 10 days following the onset of infection. On the other hand, other infectious agents may elicit only a "round cell" response. Cell-mediated forms of acute inflammation, even in very early stages, are characterized by lymphocytic infiltrate, with or without plasma cells, monocytes, and granulomata.

Besides inflammatory cells, the interstitium may be infiltrated by or contain abnormal extracellular material; this includes amyloid, immunoglobulin light chains (usually along tubular basement membranes), immune complex deposits, etc. This may be in association with similar infiltrates in glomeruli, or less commonly, may be restricted to the interstitium.

Pathogenic Mechanisms in Renal Diseases

Glomerular

Immunologic

Many glomerular and a small number of tubulo-interstitial and vascular disorders are immunologically mediated. These may be the result either of antibody-mediated or cell-mediated processes. In most instances in humans, the immediate cause or antigenic stimulus for the immune reaction is not known. The detection of antibody-mediated damage in renal tissue depends on the use of immunofluorescence microscopy.

Most glomerulopathies are immunologically mediated and are the result of antibody-induced injury. This can occur as a consequence of antibody combining with an intrinsic antigen in the glomerulus or antibody combining either in situ or in the circulation with an extrinsic glomerular antigen, with immune complexes localizing or depositing in glomeruli. With *circulating immune complexes*, the antigens may be of endogenous or exogenous origin. Endogenous antigens occur in diseases such as systemic lupus erythematosus and include components of nuclei such as DNA, histones, etc. Exogenous antigens are usually of microorganism origin and include bacterial products, hepatitis B and C viral antigens, malarial antigen, etc. Circulating immune complexes are trapped or lodge in glomeruli in the mesangium and subendothelial aspects of capillary walls. Less commonly, they may be found in subepithelial locations. It is the electron microscope that precisely localizes the deposits. Certain diseases are characterized by deposits in predominately one site, whereas other diseases may be characterized by deposits in more than one location. Once immune complexes are deposited, complement is fixed and often leukocyte infiltration follows. The white blood cells accumulate in capillary lumina and infiltrate into the mesangium; in addition, intrinsic mesangial cells may divide and may also extend into peripheral capillary walls. The leukocytes, in part, may be responsible for removal of deposited immune complexes. The names of the many glomerular disorders, diagnostic criteria, and prognostic and therapeutic implications depend on the correct localization and identification of the immune complexes in the glomeruli.

The other mechanism of antibody-induced injury results from in situ immune complex formation. This can occur in two major situations. The antibody can be directed against an intrinsic component of the glomerulus such as a portion of the basement membrane or perhaps, as shown in experimental animals, a cellular component. Alternatively, antigen may arrive in the glomerulus from the circulation and be planted or trapped in a particular location. Antibody binds with the trapped antigen, forming immune complex locally.

In humans, antibody directed against the basement membrane component is known as antiglomerular basement membrane antibody. The pattern of fluorescence is of *linear* binding of the antibody to the basement membrane. Planted antigens and glomerular epithelial cell antigen in experimental animals, when combined with antibody in situ, result in a pattern of *granular* fluorescence similar to glomeruli with deposition of circulating immune complexes.

Cell-mediated immune injury in human renal disease is evident in acute interstitial disorders such as drug-induced acute interstitial nephritis and certain forms of transplant rejection. On the other hand, cell-mediated immune mechanisms in glomerular disease are postulated with sound experimental and clinical reasoning.

Complement components, especially C5b-C9, may have a large role in producing structural and functional damage, especially in glomeruli. Recent and continuing evidence has documented the important roles of cytokines especially IL-1 and TNF as well as platelet-derived growth factor (PDGF) and transforming growth factor-β (TGF-β) in the genesis and progression of glomerular disease.

Nonimmunologic

There are several important mechanisms that result in significant glomerular damage in a wide variety of circumstances that merit comment here.

Damage to glomerular visceral epithelial cells, from a wide variety of influences, causes cell swelling with loss of individual foot processes. Further damage results in vacuolization, accumulation of protein in lysosomes (protein reabsorption droplets), and detachment of cells from the basement membrane.

With significant loss of functioning nephrons, the remnant nephrons undergo hypertrophy. While initially an adaptive process, these changes are associated with the ultimate development of segmental glomerulosclerosis, diminution in glomerular filtration, and heavy proteinuria.

Tubular and Interstitial Injury

Pathogenic mechanisms in tubulo-interstitial injury include immunologic processes (antibody-mediated and cell-mediated immunity) with cytokine expression and release, and action of inflammatory mediators. Chronic changes (interstitial fibrosis and tubular atrophy) are also the result of cytokine (PDGF and TGF-β) and complement (C5) fibroblast chemoattraction and of interaction of fibroblasts with metalloproteinases and IL-1, TNF-α, and epidermal growth factor. Fibroblasts produce collagen types I, III, IV, V; tubular cells are capable of synthesizing types I and III collagens as well as type IV (basement membrane) collagen.

Vasculature

In general, the renal arteries and arterioles respond to injuries in a manner similar to other vascular beds. However, the kidneys are frequent targets of vascular injury because of their high blood flow (approximately 25% of cardiac output); furthermore, kidney function is critically dependent on blood pressure and flow and any interference to either may have profound effects.

The major lesions affecting renal vasculature include (1) thrombosis and embolization; (2) fibrin deposition in the walls of arteries, arterioles, and glomerular capillaries; (3) inflammation and necrosis of vascular walls; and (4) arteriosclerosis. The basic pathologic features of these injuries are little different from those of vessels in other organs and tissues, and a comprehensive consideration, therefore, is not warranted except in lesions unique to renal vessels.

Perhaps the most important of these features is the vascular picture resulting from platelet activation and mural fibrin deposition. These result in different abnormalities in different-sized vessels. In small (interlobular) arteries, there is smooth muscle cell proliferation with intimal ingrowth of these cells and marked luminal narrowing. Fibrin in arteriolar walls is associated with endothelial damage and local thrombosis, often with extension of the thrombi into glomeruli. In these structures (glomeruli), endothelial cells are swollen, capillary walls are thickened with accumulation of fibrin beneath endothelial cells, and mesangial regions widened also because of fibrin deposition. Structural consequences include capillary microaneurysm formation. Healing results in varying degrees of mesangial sclerosis (increased matrix) and capillary wall double contours (1–6).

References

1. Cohen AH, Nast CC. The kidney. In: Damjanov I, Linder J, eds. Anderson's Pathology, 10th ed. St. Louis: Mosby, 1996:2071–2137.
2. Jennette JC, Olson JL, Schwartz MM, Silva FG, eds. Heptinstall's Pathology of the Kidney, 5th ed. Philadelphia: Lippincott-Raven, 1998.
3. Silva FG, D'Agati VD, Nadasdy T. Renal Biopsy Interpretation. New York: Churchill Livingstone, 1996.
4. Churg J, Bernstein J, Glassock RJ, eds. Renal Disease: Classification and Atlas of Glomerular Diseases, 2nd ed. New York: Igaku-Shoin, 1995.
5. Seshan SV, D'Agati, Appel GA, Churg J. Renal Disease: Classification and Atlas of Tubulo-Interstitial and Vascular Diseases. Baltimore: Williams & Wilkins, 1999.
6. Kern WF, Silva FG, Laszik ZG, Bane BL, Nadasdy T, Pitha JV. Atlas of Renal Pathology. Philadelphia: WB Saunders, 1999.

Section II
Glomerular Diseases with Nephrotic Syndrome Presentations

2
Membranous Glomerulopathy

Jan A. Bruijn

Introduction/Clinical Setting

Membranous glomerulopathy is a major cause of the nephrotic syndrome in adults (1,2). Only in the past decades has it been surpassed by focal and segmental glomerulosclerosis as the main cause of the nephrotic syndrome (3–5). Membranous glomerulopathy develops mostly idiopathically, but can also be seen in relation with and possibly secondary to, among others, hepatitis B, Sjögren's syndrome, transplantation, lupus erythematosus, diabetes mellitus, sarcoidosis, syphilis, exposure to certain drugs and heavy metals (penicillamine, bucillamine, gold, mercuric chloride), and malignancies (10%), including carcinomas, carcinoids, sarcomas, lymphoma's, and leukemias (2,6–10). The possibility of a malignancy must be considered especially in older patients with membranous glomerulopathy. In these patients it is also imperative to perform urinary immunoelectrophoresis routinely to rule out myeloma and renal primary amyloidosis (AL) (2). Finally, idiopathic membranous glomerulopathy, of which an autoimmune origin has not been established, must be distinguished from membranous lupus glomerulonephritis (11), as discussed in Chapter 8. Synonyms for membranous glomerulopathy are membranous nephritis, (epi)membranous nephropathy, extramembranous glomerulopathy, and perimembranous nephropathy (7,12).

Membranous glomerulopathy occurs mostly in adults with a peak incidence in the fourth and fifth decades; at all ages men are more often affected than women. Patients present most often with a nephrotic syndrome, sometimes with asymptomatic proteinuria or hematuria. The prognosis seems to be related to the level of proteinuria at presentation. In general the prognosis is excellent in children, whereas in adults 10-year patient survival is around 75%. In secondary forms the underlying disease determines the prognosis. Still, a reported fraction of around 30% of patients with membranous glomerulopathy develop chronic renal failure with depression of the glomerular filtration rate (GFR) (13). The therapeutic approach to patients with membranous glomerulopathy is still controversial (14–19).

Pathologic Findings

Light Microscopy

Morphologic changes in membranous glomerulopathy are usually present in all glomeruli found in a biopsy, with little variation in the severity of the lesions between glomeruli. Morphologic lesions, however, can differ between patients, or between biopsies taken from one patient at different time points. This is caused by the evolutionary pathologic changes occurring in the glomerular capillary walls in the course of time. These morphologic changes can be very subtle and sometimes hardly or not at all visible. This illustrates the need of performing immunofluorescence and electron microscopic studies.

In typical cases the glomerular capillary wall is diffusely thickened in different stains, as a result of the presence of nonargyrophilic, subepithelially localized immune deposits. In the methenamine-silver staining in early stages a somewhat rough aspect of the glomerular capillary walls is seen, which is not specific for membranous glomerulopathy. Irregular thickenings at the outer side of the glomerular basement membrane grow around the immune deposits and appear in the silver staining as "spikes" (Fig. 2.1). These are at first small and segmental, but they grow in the course of the disease, while they may broaden toward their end (club-shaped), embracing the deposits. Three-dimensionally they are in fact "craters," as can be well observed at places where the capillary wall is cut tangentially. As mentioned before, spike formation results from the presence of subepithelial deposits, which trigger the epithelial cells to increase their production of extracellular matrix, especially laminin (20).

In membranous glomerulopathy, due to the glomerular protein leak, the tubules often show epithelial protein resorption droplets and there may be

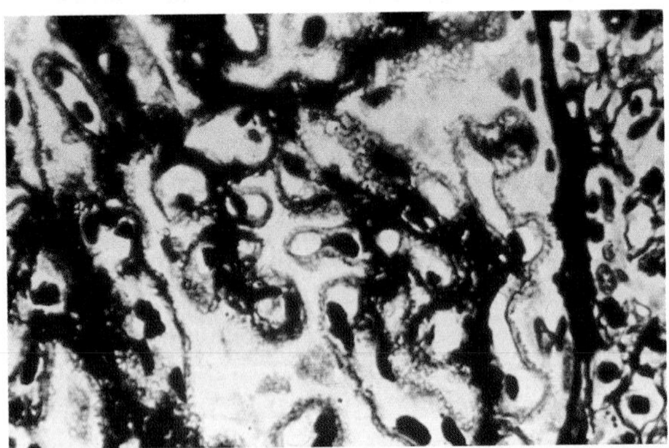

FIGURE 2.1. Glomerulus showing thickening of glomerular basement membrane (GBM) and subepithelial "spikes" in membranous glomerulopathy (silver-methenamine stain).

protein cylinders. Foam cells may be present in the interstitium or between tubular epithelial cells and are related to the hyperlipidemia and reabsorption of filtered lipoproteins, as can be seen also in nephrotic syndrome due to other causes. With progression of the glomerular lesions, nephron loss and interstitial fibrosis may occur. In late stages the glomeruli show nonspecific global sclerosis. Interstitial vessels show mostly no abnormalities in membranous glomerulopathy. The extent of interstitial damage correlates strongly with prognosis (21).

Immunofluorescence Microscopy

Immunofluorescence investigations in membranous glomerulopathy generally reveal granular deposits of immune reactants, which follow the contours of the glomerular basement membrane. Immuno-electron microscopical studies have shown that these immune reactants are present in the electron dense deposits described above. The deposits can sometimes be very finely granular, which may lead to the immunofluorescence pattern being falsely interpreted as linear. Deposits in the mesangium are absent in most cases. The most often occurring component in the immune deposits is immunoglobulin G (IgG) (Fig. 2.2). In addition, C3 is often found, while IgM and IgA have been found in about half of the published cases. When in addition to IgG, IgM, and C3 also IgA and C1q are found ("full

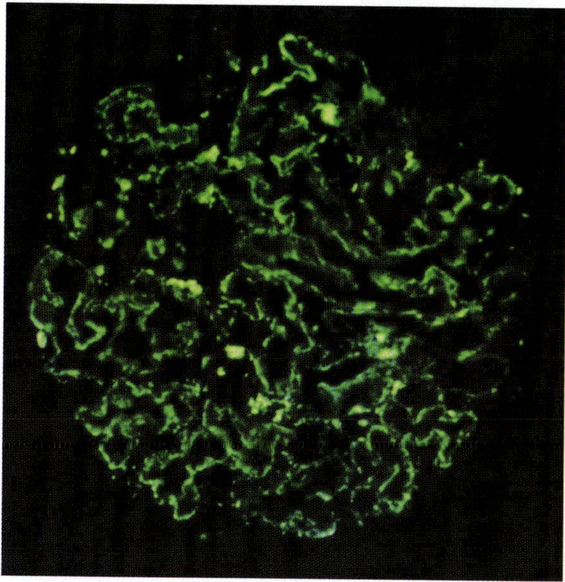

FIGURE 2.2. Immunofluorescence showing diffuse fine granular distribution pattern of immunoglobulin G (IgG) along the GBM in membranous glomerulopathy.

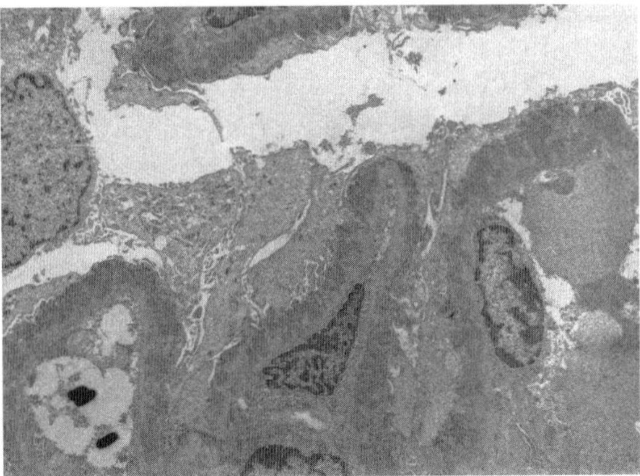

FIGURE 2.3. Electron microscopy showing subepithelial electron dense deposits, spike formation of GBM and obliteration of visceral epithelial cell pedicles in membranous glomerulopathy.

house"), suspicion of lupus membranous glomerulopathy should arise (22).

Electron Microscopy

At electron microscopy the spikes can most often be found in different stages of development, between and around the electron dense deposits (Fig. 2.3). As described, the immune deposits in membranous nephropathy are localized subepithelially and sometimes intramembranously. The subepithelial deposits are in contact with the glomerular epithelial cells. In these cells the cytoplasm close to the deposits often shows fibrillary condensation, while there is extensive obliteration of the pedicles. The epithelial cells may also show reabsorption droplets and microvillous transformation. The electron dense deposits show most often a finely granular ultrastructure. The surrounding spikes vary in size and shape, suggesting a certain sequence of events. With increasing basement membrane pathology the immunopathologic evidence for the presence of immune complexes decreases, as does the protein secretion. The size of the electron dense deposits and the thickness of the basement membranes are significantly correlated with clinical parameters such as proteinuria, serum creatinine, and creatinine clearance, and with prognosis (23,24).

Etiology/Pathogenesis

Membranous glomerulopathy is a morphologic diagnosis. It describes a disease characterized by a spectrum of changes in the glomerular capillary wall, initiated by the formation of subepithelial immune complexes. It is assumed that immunologic pathogenetic mechanisms underlie membranous glomerulopathy, as reviewed extensively elsewhere (6,25–29). Membranous glomerulopathy is an immune complex disease associated with a T-helper 2 (Th2) nephritogenic immune response and overproduction of interleukin-4 (IL-4), a principal Th2 cytokine (30). Observations from animal models and some in humans suggest that the production of antibodies directed at glycoproteins occurring on the visceral epithelial cell surface results in in situ formation of subepithelial immune complexes and glomerular damage (7,25,29,31–33). As discussed in more detail in the paragraph on membranous lupus nephritis, (Chapter 8), the purely subepithelial location of the immune complexes in membranous nephropathy leads to complement activation, but not to chemotaxis and activation of inflammatory cells with subsequent glomerular cell proliferation, since inflammatory cells cannot pass the glomerular basement membrane. Indeed, glomerular proliferation and influx of inflammatory cells are usually absent in membranous glomerulopathy. For this reason, the term *membranous glomerulonephritis* is regarded by some as a misnomer that should be replaced by the term *membranous glomerulopathy*. Subepithelial formation of immune complexes leads to podocyte damage with compensatory alterations in the expression of podocyte-associated molecules such as nephrin (34). In experimental membranous glomerulopathy, the onset of proteinuria is coincident with complement-dependent alterations in the association of nephrin with the actin cytoskeleton and loss of podocyte slit-diaphragm integrity (35). This leads to foot process broadening and depression of the single-nephron ultrafiltration coefficient and decrease of the GFR early in the course of the disease (36). Subepithelial deposits in membranous nephropathy drive glomerular epithelial cells to diminish their expression of vascular endothelial growth factor (VEGF), a presumably protective cytokine (37), and increase that of transforming growth factor-β1 (TGF-β1). In turn, TGF-β1 dysregulates the expression of matrix genes, leading to production of quantitatively and qualitatively abnormal basement membrane matrix by the glomerular visceral epithelial cells (38). This would somehow lead to both increased permeability of the glomerular basement membrane and ensuing nephrotic syndrome, and to the formation of spikes that contain predominantly laminin (20). Indeed, proteinuria in membranous glomerulopathy seems to result mainly from a loss of size selectivity of the glomerular capillary walls, in contrast to the defect in, for example, minimal change glomerulopathy, which results mainly from a loss of charge selectivity (2). In those patients with membranous nephropathy who develop chronic renal failure with further depression of GFR, hypofiltration is the consequence of a biphasic loss of glomerular ultrafiltration capacity, initially owing to impaired hydraulic permeability that is later exacerbated by a superimposed loss of functioning glomeruli and of filtration surface area (13). Severe proteinuria seems to be the main factor responsible for the upregulation of fibrogenic cytokines in tubular epithelial cells (39).

Clinicopathologic Correlations

The natural history of the untreated disease is variable. Complete or partial spontaneous remissions of proteinuria eventually occur in 40% to 50% of patients, usually accompanied by stable renal function (21). The remainder slowly progress to end-stage renal disease or die of complications or from unrelated disorder after 5 to 15 years (21). Factors influencing the progression of membranous glomerulopathy are numerous and include age, renal function, and albuminuria at the onset, and interactions between gene polymorphisms, such as those of nitric oxide synthase and the renin-angiotensin system (21,40). Membranous glomerulopathy may be complicated by focal and segmental glomerulosclerosis including the collapsing variant, also in HIV-negative patients (41).

The treatment of membranous glomerulopathy remains both controversial and suboptimal. For those patients who have persistent nephrotic proteinuria or manifest loss of renal function, steroids and immunosuppressive drugs are used (42). Angiotensin II inhibition may slow progression by controlling proteinuria (42). Alternative therapies and future intervention modalities include vaccines, inhibitors of plasminogen activator, humanized monoclonal antibodies, mycophenolate mofetil, and pentoxifylline (43). Treatment of secondary membranous glomerulopathy generally targets the primary diseases rather than the renal lesion (44). Recent data obtained from animal models suggest that antibody binding in membranous glomerulopathy depends on the conformation of the antigenic target sequence, and that interference with the immunologic basis of the disease by use of synthetic peptides should be possible (45–47).

The sequence of events occurring during the development of membranous glomerulopathy is so constant that its course can be divided into several stages (48). In stage I light microscopic changes are absent, but immunofluorescence shows granular aggregates of immunoglobulins. In stage II spikes are present, which in stage III embrace the subepithelial aggregates. This is accompanied by obliteration of pedicles. Stage IV is characterized by variation in electron density of the deposits and severe thickening and deformation of the glomerular basement membrane. In general, a relation exists between the morphologic stage of the disease and the clinical severity and duration. Interestingly, in patients in remission reversibility of the morphologic lesion has been reported (49). Of note, novel molecular biologic techniques may allow further subclassification as well as more accurate determination of the prognosis (50,51).

References

1. Lewis EJ. Management of the nephrotic syndrome in adults. In: Cameron JS, Glassock RJ, eds. The Nephrotic Syndrome. New York: Marcel Dekker, 1988:461–521.

2. Orth SR, Ritz E. The nephrotic syndrome. N Engl J Med 338:1202–1211, 1998.
3. Haas M, Spargo BH, Coventry S. Increasing incidence of focal-segmental glomerulosclerosis among adult nephropathies: a 20-year renal biopsy study. Am J Kidney Dis 26:740–750, 1995.
4. D'Agati V. The many masks of focal segmental glomerulosclerosis. Kidney Int 46:1223–1241, 1994.
5. Braden GL, Mulhern JG, O'Shea MH, Nash SV, Ucci AA, Germain MJ. Changing incidence of glomerular diseases in adults. Am J Kidney Dis 35:878–883, 2000.
6. Hricik DE, Chung-Park M, Sedor JR. Glomerulonephritis. N Engl J Med 339:888–900, 1998.
7. Schwartz MM. Membranous glomerulonephritis. In: Jennette JC, Olson JL, Schwartz MM, Silva FG, eds. Heptinstall's Pathology of the Kidney, 5th ed. Philadelphia: Lippincott, 1998:259–308.
8. Luyckx C, Van DB, Vanrenterghem Y, Maes B. Carcinoid tumor and membranous glomerulonephritis: coincidence or malignancy-associated glomerulonephritis? Clin Nephrol 57:80–84, 2002.
9. Nagahama K, Matsushita H, Hara M, Ubara Y, Hara S, Yamada A. Bucillamine induces membranous glomerulonephritis. Am J Kidney Dis 39:706–712, 2002.
10. Strippoli GF, Manno C, Rossini M, Occhiogrosso G, Maiorano E, Schena FP. Primary cerebral lymphoma and membranous nephropathy: a still unreported association. Am J Kidney Dis 39:E22, 2002.
11. Haas M, Zikos D. Membranous nephropathy. Distinction of latent membranous lupus nephritis from idiopathic membranous nephropathy on renal biopsy. Pathol Case Rev 3:175–179, 1998.
12. Schwartz MM. Membranous glomerulonephritis. In: Heptinstall RH, ed. Pathology of the Kidney, 4th ed. Boston, Little, Brown, 1992:559–626.
13. Squarer A, Lemley KV, Ambalavanan S, et al. Mechanisms of progressive glomerular injury in membranous nephropathy. J Am Soc Nephrol 9:1389–1398, 1998.
14. Polenakovik MH, Grcevska L. Treatment and long-term follow-up of patients with stage II to III idiopathic membranous nephropathy. Am J Kidney Dis 34:911–917, 1999.
15. Ruggenenti P, Mosconi L, Vendramin G, et al. ACE inhibition improves glomerular size selectivity in patients with idiopathic membranous nephropathy and persistent nephrotic syndrome. Am J Kidney Dis 35:381–391, 2000.
16. Geddes CC, Cattran DC. The treatment of idiopathic membranous nephropathy. Semin Nephrol 20:299–308, 2000.
17. Branten AJW, Wetzels JFM. Short- and long-term efficacy of oral cyclophosphamide and steroids in patients with membranous nephropathy and renal insufficiency. Clin Nephrol 56:1–9, 2001.
18. Remuzzi G, Chiurchiu C, Abbate M, Brusegan V, Bontempelli M, Ruggenenti P. Rituximab for idiopathic membranous nephropathy. Lancet 360:923–924, 2002.
19. Cattran DC. Membranous nephropathy: quo vadis? Kidney Int 61:349–350, 2002.

20. Fukatsu A, Matsuo S, Killen PD, Martin GR, Andres GA, Brentjens JR. The glomerular distribution of type IV collagen and laminin in human membranous glomerulonephritis. Hum Pathol 19:64–68, 1990.
21. Glassock RJ. Diagnosis and natural course of membranous nephropathy. Semin Nephrol 23:324–332, 2003.
22. Picken MM. The role of kidney biopsy in the management of patients with systemic lupus erythematosus. Pathol Case Rev 3:204–209, 1998.
23. Tóth T, Takebayashi S. Idiopathic membranous glomerulonephritis: a clinicopathologic and quantitative morphometric study. Clin Nephrol 38:14–19, 1992.
24. Yoshimoto K, Yokoyama H, Wada T, et al. Pathologic findings of initial biopsies reflect the outcomes of membranous nephropathy. Kidney Int 65:148–153, 2004.
25. Bruijn JA, Hoedemaeker PJ. Nephritogenic immune reactions involving native renal antigens. In: Massry SG, Glassock RJ, eds. Textbook of Nephrology, 3rd ed. Baltimore: Williams & Wilkins, 1995:627–631.
26. Bruijn JA, de Heer E, Hoedemaeker PJ. Immune mechanisms in injury to glomeruli and tubulo-interstitial tissue. In: Jones TC, ed. Monographs on Pathology of Laboratory Animals. Urinary System, 2nd ed. New York: Springer-Verlag, 1998:199–224.
27. de Heer E, Bruijn JA, Hoedemaeker PJ. Heymann nephritis revisited. New insights into the pathogenesis of experimental membranous glomerulonephritis. Clin Exp Immunol 94:393–394, 1993.
28. Maruyama S, Cantu E, Demartino C, et al. Membranous glomerulonephritis induced in the pig by antibody to angiotensin-converting enzyme: considerations on its relevance to the pathogenesis of human idiopathic membranous glomerulonephritis. J Am Soc Nephrol 10:2102–2108, 1999.
29. Cattran DC. Idiopathic membranous glomerulonephritis. Kidney Int 59: 1983–1994, 2001.
30. Masutani K, Taniguchi M, Nakashima H, et al. Up-regulated interleukin-4 production by peripheral T-helper cells in idiopathic membranous nephropathy. Nephrol Dial Transplant 19:580–586, 2004.
31. Van Leer EHG, de Roo GM, Bruijn JA, Hoedemaeker PJ, de Heer E. Synergistic effects of anti-gp330 and anti-dipeptidyl peptidase type IV antibodies in the induction of glomerular damage. Exp Nephrol 1:292–300, 1993.
32. Oleinikov AV, Feliz BJ, Makker SP. A small N-terminal 60-kD fragment of gp600 (Megalin), the major autoantigen of active Heymann nephritis, can indiuce a full-blown disease. J Am Soc Nephrol 11:57–64, 2000.
33. Debiec H, Guigonis V, Mougenot B, et al. Antenatal membranous glomerulonephritis due to anti-neutral endopeptidase antibodies. N Engl J Med 346: 2053–2060, 2002.
34. Koop K, Eikmans M, Baelde HJ, et al. Expression of podocyte-associated molecules in acquired human kidney diseases. J Am Soc Nephrol 14:2063–2071, 2003.
35. Saran AM, Yuan H, Takeuchi E, McLaughlin M, Salant DJ. Complement mediates nephrin redistribution and actin dissociation in experimental membranous nephropathy. Kidney Int 64:2072–2078, 2003.

36. Hladunewich MA, Lemley KV, Blouch KL, Myers BD. Determinants of GFR depression in early membranous nephropathy. Am J Physiol Renal Physiol 284:F1014–F1022, 2003.
37. Honkanen E, von Willebrand E, Koskinen P, et al. Decreased expression of vascular endothelial growth factor in idiopathic membranous glomerulonephritis: relationships to clinical course. Am J Kidney Dis 42:1139–1148, 2003.
38. Kim TS, Kim JY, Hong HK, Lee HS. mRNA expression of glomerular basement membrane proteins and TGF-β1 in human membranous nephropathy. J Pathol 189:425–430, 1999.
39. Mezzano SA, Droguett MA, Burgos ME, et al. Overexpression of chemokines, fibrogenic cytokines, and myofibroblasts in human membranous nephropathy. Kidney Int 57:147–158, 2000.
40. Stratta P, Bermond F, Guarrera S, et al. Interaction between gene polymorphisms of nitric oxide synthase and renin-angiotensin system in the progression of membranos glomerulonephritis. Nephrol Dial Transplant 19:587–595, 2004.
41. Al-Shamari A, Yeung K, Levin A, Taylor P, Magil A. Collapsing glomerulopathy coexisting with membranous glomerulonephritis in native kidney biopsies: a report of 3 HIV-negative patients. Am J Kidney Dis 42:591–595, 2003.
42. Schieppati A, Ruggenenti P, Perna A, Remuzzi G. Nonimmunosuppressive therapy of membranous nephropathy. Semin Nephrol 23:333–339, 2003.
43. Kshirsagar AV, Nachman PH, Falk RJ. Alternative therapies and future intervention for treatment of membranous nephropathy. Semin Nephrol 23:362–372, 2003.
44. Jefferson JA, Couser WG. Therapy of membranous nephropathy associated with malignancy and secondary causes. Semin Nephrol 23:400–405, 2003.
45. Luca ME, Van der Wal A, Paul L, Bruijn JA, de Heer E. Treatment with mycophenolate mofetil attenuates the development of Heymann nephritis. Exp Nephrol 8:77–83, 2000.
46. Luca ME, de Geus B, Sahali D, Bruijn JA, Verroust P, de Heer E. Isolation of cDNAs encoding immunogenic regions of gp330, the autoantigen involved in Heymann nephritis. Clin Exp Immunol 104:312–317, 1996.
47. Kerjaschki D, Ullrich R, Exner M, Orlando RA, Farquhar MG. Induction of passive Heymann nephritis with antibodies specific for a synthetic peptide derived from the receptor-associated protein. J Exp Med 183:2007–2015, 1996.
48. Ehrenreich T, Churg J. Pathology of membranous nephropathy. In: Sommers SC, ed. Pathology Annual 1968, vol 3. New York: Appleton-Century-Crofts, 1968:145–154.
49. Gonzalo A, Mampaso F, Barcena R, Gallego N, Ortuno J. Membranous nephropathy associated with hepatitis B virus infection: long-term clinical and histological outcome. Nephrol Dial Transplant 14:416–418, 1999.
50. Eikmans M, Baelde JJ, de Heer E, Bruijn JA. RNA expression profiling as prognostic tool in renal patients: toward nephrogenomics. Kidney Int 62:1125–1135, 2002.
51. Eikmans M, Baelde HJ, Hagen EC, et al. Renal mRNA levels as prognostic tools in kidney diseases. J Am Soc Nephrol 14:899–907, 2003.

3 Membranoproliferative Glomerulonephritis

Agnes B. Fogo

Introduction/Clinical Setting

Membranoproliferative glomerulonephritis (MPGN) refers to a pattern of injury characterized by diffuse mesangial expansion due to endocapillary proliferation and increased mesangial matrix, and thickened capillary walls, often with a split "tram-track" appearance (1,2). The immune complexes may be undefined in terms of the inciting antigen ("idiopathic") or secondary to chronic infections (3). Of note, basement membrane splitting may be seen in other non–immune complex injuries, such as the late phase of thrombotic microangiopathy (3). Although light microscopy may appear similar to MPGN, immunofluorescence findings and electron microscopy readily allow recognition of the immune complexes in MPGN. We and others prefer to use the term *membranoproliferative glomerulonephritis* only for immune complex glomerulonephritides with this pattern (1). Membranoproliferative glomerulonephritis type I typically presents as combined nephritic/nephrotic syndrome with hypocomplementemia. Patients typically have progressive renal disease, with about 50% renal survival at 10 years in children, and similar rates of progression in adults. Idiopathic MPGN is more common in children and young adults, whereas MPGN-type lesions are more commonly secondary to chronic infections in adults. New insights into the role of complement regulation in renal injury are adding to our understanding of the etiology of injury in cases previously classified as idiopathic.

Pathologic Findings

Light Microscopy

Membranoproliferative glomerulonephritis has been divided into three types. Type I characteristically has subendothelial deposits, resulting in a thickened capillary wall and a double contour of the glomerular basement membrane (GBM) by silver stains, and endocapillary proliferation (1,4).

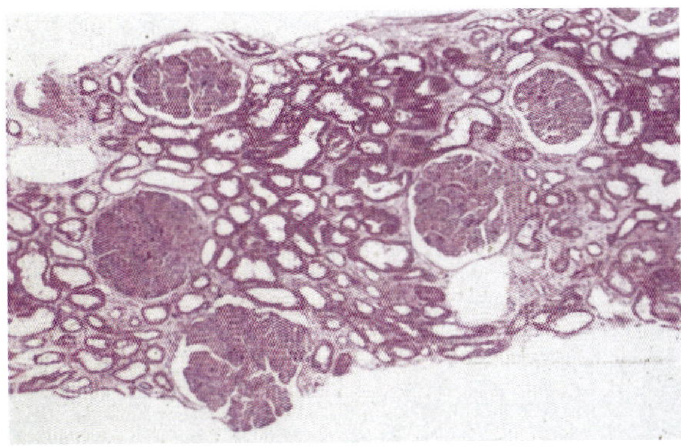

FIGURE 3.1. Lobular appearance due to diffuse, global endocapillary proliferation of all glomeruli in membranoproliferative glomerulonephritis (MPGN) type I [periodic acid-Schiff (PAS)].

This appearance results from so-called circumferential mesangial interposition, whereby mesangial cells, infiltrating mononuclear cells, or even portions of endothelial cells interpose themselves between the endothelium and the basement membrane, with new, inner basement membrane being laid down (5). A circumferential, or partial, double contour basement membrane results. Of note, in non–immune complex diseases with splitting seen by light microscopy (e.g., transplant glomerulopathy, chronic injury after hemolytic uremic syndrome), electron microscopy shows that the double contour results from widening of the GBM due to increased lucency of the lamina rara interna with new basement membrane formed underneath the endothelium. In MPGN type I, the glomeruli show endocapillary proliferation with increased mesangial cellularity and matrix, and lobular simplification (Figs. 3.1 to 3.3). The term *mesangiocapillary glo-*

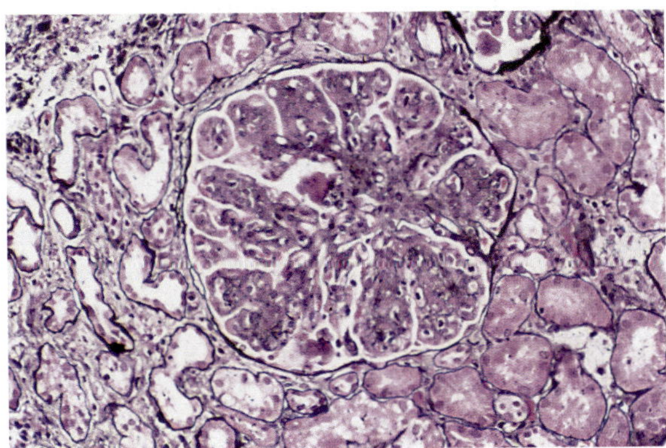

FIGURE 3.2. Diffuse, global endocapillary proliferation with extensive glomerular basement membrane (GBM) splitting in MPGN type I (Jones silver stain).

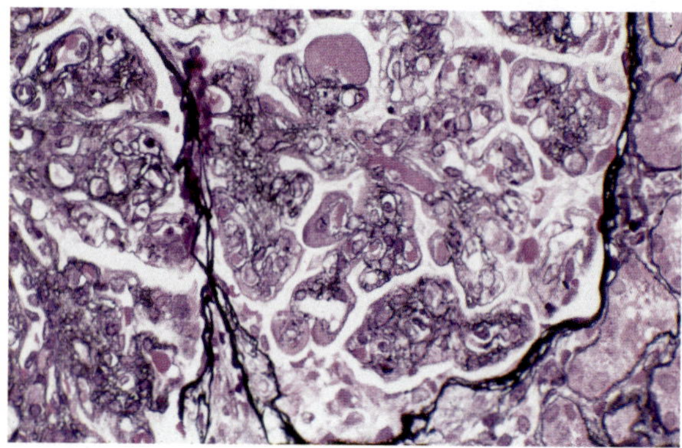

FIGURE 3.3. Diffuse, global endocapillary proliferation with GBM splitting and visible large subendothelial deposits in MPGN type I (Jones silver stain).

merulonephritis has also been used for MPGN type I. Increased mononuclear cells and occasional neutrophils may be present. The proliferation is typically uniform and diffuse in idiopathic MPGN, contrasting the irregular involvement most commonly seen in proliferative lupus nephritis (Fig. 3.1). In secondary forms of MPGN, the injury may be more irregular. Crescents may occur in both idiopathic and secondary forms. Deposits do not involve extraglomerular sites. Lesions progress with less cellularity and more pronounced matrix accumulation and sclerosis over time (6). Tubular and vascular fibrosis and sclerosis proportional to glomerular scarring are seen late in the course.

Dense deposit disease (DDD), also called MPGN type II, is a separate disease entity from MPGN type I. Due to its similar light microscopic appearance, it conventionally has been classified with MPGN (7). It is much rarer than type I, accounting for 15% to 35% of total MPGN cases. By light microscopy, endocapillary proliferation is present. The basement membranes are thickened and highly refractile and eosinophilic, with involved areas with strings of deposits looking like a string of sausages. The deposits are periodic acid-Schiff (PAS) positive and stain brown with silver stain. Thickening also affects tubular basement membranes and Bowman's capsule. Crescents may be present.

Membranoproliferative glomerulonephritis type III shows, in addition to the subendothelial and mesangial deposits, numerous subepithelial deposits. It may not, however, represent an entity separate from MPGN type I (8,9). Although C3 nephritic factor is rarely found in these patients, clinical distinction of this morphology has not been apparent.

Immunofluorescence Microscopy

The immunofluorescence findings are variable in MPGN type I. Typically, immunoglobulin G (IgG) and IgM and C3 are present in an irregular capil-

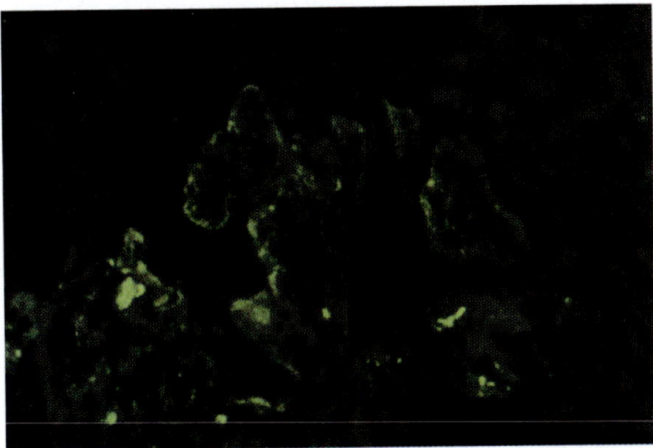

FIGURE 3.4. Coarsely granular capillary loop and mesangial deposits in MPGN [anti–immunoglobulin G (IgG) antibody immunofluorescence].

lary and mesangial distribution (Fig. 3.4). Immunoglobulin A (IgA) is present in only a small proportion of cases. Of note, C3 staining may be dominant, and staining for immunoglobulin may even be lost, especially in secondary MPGN.

In DDD, C3 staining outlines the capillary wall, and may be smooth, granular, or discontinuous. Mesangial bright granular staining can be present. Immunoglobulin is usually not detected, indicating the dense deposits are not classic antigen-antibody immune complexes. However, segmental IgM or less often IgG and very rarely IgA have been reported (10).

Electron Microscopy

By electron microscopy, MPGN type I shows numerous dense deposits in subendothelial and mesangial areas (Fig. 3.5). Vague wormy or microtu-

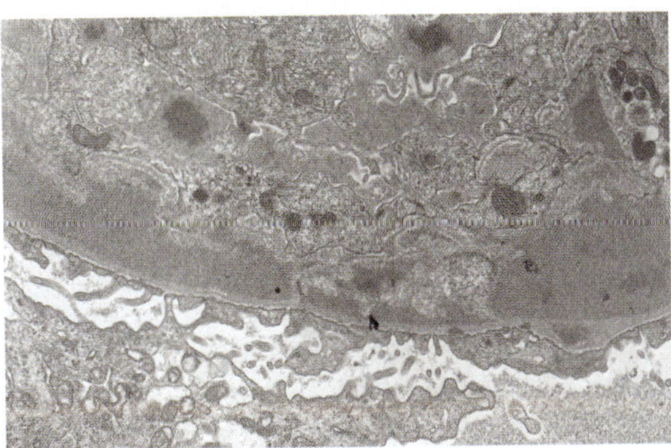

FIGURE 3.5. Subendothelial immune complex deposits in MPGN type I (electron microscopy).

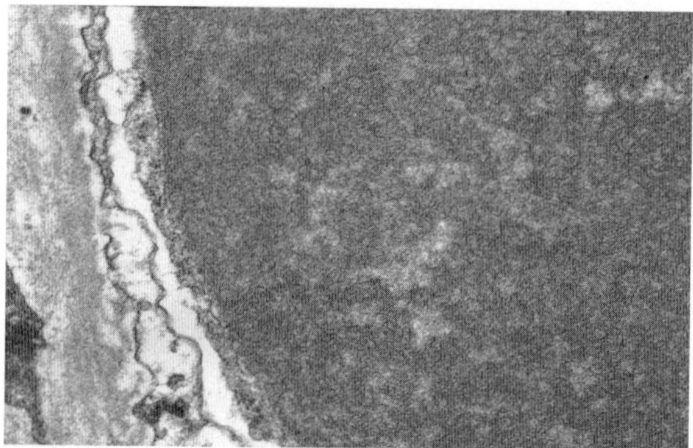

FIGURE 3.6. Intracapillary deposits with vague, short fibrillary substruture, in MPGN caused by hepatitis C–associated cryoglobulin (electron microscopy).

bular substructure suggests a possible cryoglobulin component (Fig. 3.6). So-called mesangial interposition is detected (Fig. 3.7), which refers to the interposition of cytoplasmic processes of mononuclear cells between the endothelial cell and the basement membrane. The precise origin of the interposing cells has not been directly proven, and they may in fact be derived from mononuclear inflammatory cells. Reduplication of new basement material is present immediately under the swollen endothelial cells, resulting in the splitting visualized by light microscopy by silver stains (1,4).

The lamina densa of the basement membrane in DDD shows a very dense transformation without discrete immune complex-type deposits

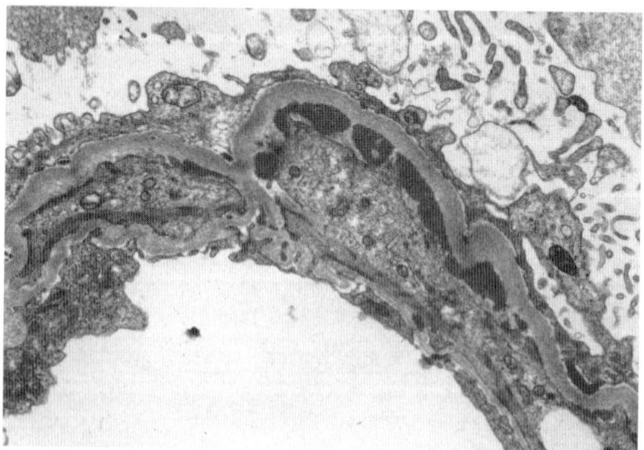

FIGURE 3.7. Subendothelial deposits with underlying interposed cell (so-called mesangial interposition) and underlying new GBM formation, resulting in split appearance by light microscopy in MPGN (electron microscopy).

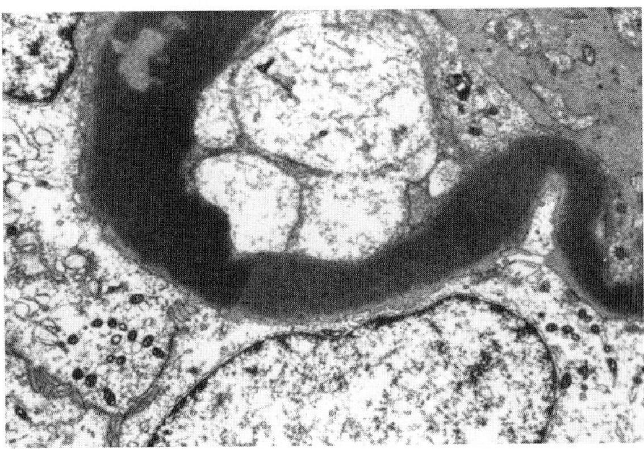

FIGURE 3.8. Dense transformation of the GBM in dense deposit disease (electron microscopy).

(Fig. 3.8) (7,11). Similar dense material is often found in the mesangial areas in addition to increased matrix. Increased mesangial cellularity and/or mesangial interposition are far less common than in type I MPGN. Epithelial cells show varying degrees of reactive changes, from vacuolization, to microvillous transformation, to foot process effacement. Tubular basement membranes and Bowman's capsule may show similar densities. The precise nature of the dense material is not established. However, studies support the idea that these densities represent a biochemical modification of the glycoprotein components of the normal basement membrane.

Etiology/Pathogenesis

The MPGN lesions have been recognized to occur secondary to a number of chronic infectious processes, including hepatitis B, hepatitis C, syphilis, subacute bacterial endocarditis, etc. Membranoproliferative glomerulonephritis may rarely occur due to inherited deficiency of complement, or partial lipodystrophy. If a chronic bacterial infection is causing MPGN-type lesions, hump-type subepithelial deposits may be present (see Chapter 5).

Generally, morphologic features do not allow precise classification of the underlying agent in most cases of type I MPGN. However, a large number (~25% in the United Sates) of previously idiopathic MPGN cases in adults have been associated with hepatitis C infection (12). This association was not seen in a U.S. series of children with MPGN. Morphologic features suggestive of hepatitis C with cryoglogulin as an underlying cause include vague substructure of deposits, with short, curved, vaguely fibrillar deposits (Fig. 3.6) (suggestive of mixed cryoglobulinemia), or rarely microtubular substructure, strongly PAS-positive cryo-"plugs" in capillary lumina (Fig. 3.9), vasculitis, predominant IgM deposits, sometimes with clonality (13). Cryoglobulinemia is commonly associated with hepatitis C, an RNA virus (14,15). Approximately 150,000 cases of hepatitis C infection occur per year in the United States. Of these, approximately half have liver disease, with 15,000 developing chronic active hepatitis and/or cirrhosis. The prevalence of hepatitis C infection is approximately 0.6% in the United States, reaching up to 6% in Africa. In one large series of hepatitis C–positive cases affecting the kidney, 40 patients with an average age of 46 years were studied. The most common risk factors for infection in this series were intravenous drug abuse, and blood transfusion. The mixed type 2 cryoglobulinemia associated with various infections is postulated to be due to the production of rheumatoid factor in response to complexes of IgG bound to foreign antigens (16). Hepatitis C virus RNA precipitated with cryoglobulin in serum samples from patients with type 2 mixed cryoglobulinemia, supporting a role for the virus as an antigen in the cryoglobulin (16). Cryoglobulinemia may also manifest as a more acute glomerulonephritis, and may even show strongly PAS-positive cryo-plugs (hyaline thrombi) visualized in capillary lumina (Fig. 3.9). Deposits of

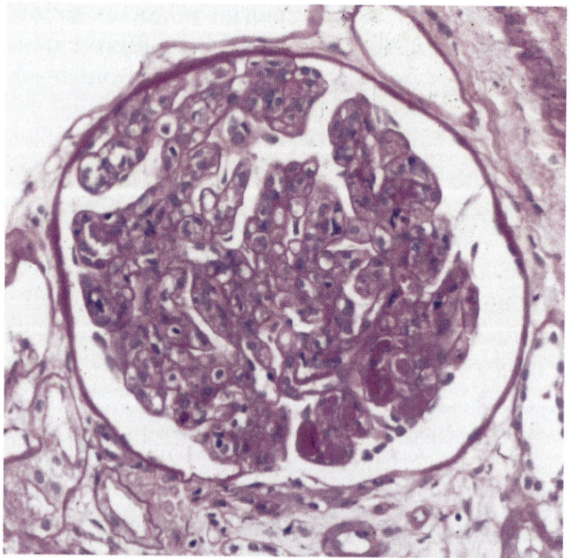

FIGURE 3.9. Global endocapillary proliferation, splitting of GBM and brightly PAS-positive so-called cryo-plugs in capillary lumina, characteristic of MPGN due to cryoglobulins (PAS).

cryoglobulin typically show vague, short, fibrillary substruture by electron microscopy (Fig. 3.6). There may also be vasculitis involving medium-sized arteries in cryoglobulinemic glomerulonephritis.

In contrast, DDD has a distinct pathogenesis related to IgG autoantibodies (C3 nephritic factor, C3NeF) directed at C3 convertase, resulting in alternate pathway complement activation. C3NeF stabilizes the C3 convertase C3bBb, resulting in alternate pathway-mediated C3 breakdown and decreased C3. Early components of the classic pathway, that is, C1q and C4, usually show normal serum levels. Sometimes DDD occurs in association with partial lipodystrophy, a condition with loss of adipose tissue, decreased complement, and the presence of C3NeF (7,17). Further, a porcine model of factor II deficiency has similarities to DDD (18). Factor H inactivates factor C3bBb. These associations have suggested that abnormal complement regulation predisposes to DDD. However, clinical measures of complement, C3NeF, or presence of partial lipodystrophy did not predict clinical outcome among patients with DDD, and some patients with MPGN type 1 also have C3NeF. Some patients with partial lipodystrophy and C3NeF do not have DDD, further indication that complement abnormalities alone are insufficient to produce the disease.

Clinicopathologic Correlations

Type I MPGN has an inexorable downhill course clinically (1,17,19). Patients present with proteinuria, which reaches nephrotic levels in two thirds. Renal disease associated with hepatitis C and cryoglobulin most often is manifest as type I MPGN, although membranous glomerulonephritis has been described. Patients with cryoglobulins often have systemic disease in addition to renal involvement (20). Necrotizing arteritis may also occur secondary to hepatitis C infection (21–23). In these patients with renal disease and hepatitis C infection, purpura is frequently present. Sixteen percent showed signs of liver disease. Tests for cryoglobulins were positive at some point of the disease course in 80% of patients. Most patients showed decreased complement (90%). Demonstration of hepatitis C in kidney tissue has not been documented directly within deposits. However, hepatitis C virus–like particles have been identified within the dense deposits, and hepatitis C virus has been isolated from renal tissue (12).

Treatment so far has offered limited success. Type I MPGN has recurred in up to 30% of transplants in some series (17). However, the disease may have a more benign clinical course when it recurs. Interferon-α therapy decreases symptoms of renal involvement in hepatitis C-associated MPGN, but relapses are prompt as soon as therapy is discontinued (12). Dense deposit disease has very frequent, near 100% morphologic recurrence in the transplant, but renal failure does not usually result (17,24).

References

1. Habib R, Kleinknecht C, Gubler MC, Levy M. Idopathic membranoproliferative glomerulonephritis in children: report of 105 cases. Clin Nephrol 1:194–214, 1973.
2. Strife CF, McEnery PT, McAdams AJ, West CD. Membranoproliferative glomerulonephritis with disruption of the glomerular basement membrane. Clin Nephrol 7:65–72, 1977.
3. Rennke HG. Nephrology forum: secondary membranoproliferative glomerulonephritis. Kidney Int 47:643–656, 1995.
4. Jones DB. Glomerulonephritis. Am J Pathol 29:33–51, 1953.
5. Katz SM. Reduplication of the glomerular basement membrane: a study of 110 cases. Arch Pathol Lab Med 105:67–70, 1981.
6. Taguchi T, Bohle A. Evaluation of change with time of glomerular morphology in membranoproliferative glomerulonephritis: a serial biopsy study of 33 cases. Clin Nephrol 31:297–306, 1989.
7. Habib R, Gubler MC, Loirat C, Maiz HB, Levy M. Dense deposit disease: a variant of membranoproliferative glomerulonephritis. Kidney Int 7:204–215, 1975.
8. Anders D, Agricola B, Sippel M, Theones W. Basement membrane changes in membranoproliferative glomerulonephritis. II. Characterization of a third type by silver impregnation of ultra thin sections: Virchows Arch [Pathol Anat] 376:1–19, 1977.
9. Strife CF, Jackson EC, McAdams AJ. Type III membranoproliferative glomerulonephritis: long-term clinical and morphological evaluation. Clin Nephrol 21:323–334, 1984.
10. Belgiojoso GB, Tarantino A, Bazzi C, Colasanti G, Guerra L, Durante A. Immunofluorescence patterns in chronic membranoproliferative glomerulonephritis (MPGN). Clin Nephrol 6:303–310, 1976.
11. Berger J, Galle P. Dépots denses au sein des membranes basales du rein: étude en microscopies optique et électronique. Presse Med 71:2351–2354, 1963.
12. Johnson RJ, Gretch DR, Yamabe H, et al. Membranoproliferative glomerulonephritis associated with hepatitis C virus infection. N Engl J Med 328: 465–470, 1993.
13. Feiner H, Gallo G. Ultrastructure in glomerulonephritis associated with cryoglobulinemia. A report of six cases and review of the literature. Am J Pathol 88:145–155, 1977.
14. Misiani R, Bellavita P, Fenili D, et al. Hepatitis C virus infection in patients with essential mixed cryoglobulinemia. Ann Intern Med 117:573–577, 1992.
15. Pascual M, Perrin L, Giostra E, Schifferli JA. Hepatitis C virus in patients with cryoglobulinemia type II. J Infect Dis 162:569–570, 1990.
16. Agnello V, Chung RT, Kaplan LM. A role for hepatitis C virus infection in type II cryoglobulinemia. N Engl J Med 327:1490–1495, 1992.
17. Cameron JS, Turner DR, Heaton J, et al. Idiopathic mesangiocapillary glomerulonephritis. Comparison of types I and II in children and adults and long-term prognosis. Am J Med 74:175–192, 1983.
18. Hegasy GA, Manuelian T, Hogasen K, Jansen JH, Zipfel PF. The molecular basis for hereditary porcine membranoproliferative glomerulonephritis type

II: point mutations in the factor H coding sequence block protein secretion. Am J Pathol 161:2027–2034, 2002.
19. Droz D, Noel LH, Barbonel C, Grünfeld JP. Long-term evolution of membranoproliferative glomerulonephritis in adults: spontaneous clinical remission in 13 cases with proven regression of glomerular lesions in 5 cases. Nephrologie 3:6–11, 1982.
20. Ferri C, Greco F, Longombardo G, et al. Association between hepatitis C virus and mixed cryoglobulinemia. Clin Exp Rheumatol 9:621–624, 1992.
21. Druet P, Letonturier P, Contet A, Mandet C. Cryoglobulinaemia in human renal diseases. A study of seventy-six cases. Clin Exp Immunol 15:483–496, 1973.
22. Perez GO, Pardo V, Fletcher MA. Renal involvement in essential mixed cryoglobulinemia. Am J Kidney Dis 10:276–280, 1987.
23. Tarantino A, De Vecchi A, Montagnino G, et al. Renal disease in essential mixed cryoglobulinaemia. Q J Med 50:1–30, 1981.
24. Andresdottir MB, Assmann KJ, Hoitsma AJ, et al. Renal transplantation in patients with dense deposit disease: morphological characteristics of recurrent disease and clinical outcome. Nephrol Dial Transplant 14:1723–1731, 1999.

4
Minimal Change Disease and Focal Segmental Glomerulosclerosis

Agnes B. Fogo

Introduction/Clinical Setting

Minimal change disease (MCD) and focal segmental glomerulosclerosis (FSGS) are both common causes of the nephrotic syndrome. Minimal change disease accounts for greater than 90% of cases of nephrotic syndrome in children, vs. 10% to 15% of adults with nephrotic syndrome (1). Focal segmental glomerulosclerosis has been increasing in incidence in the United States in both African Americans and in Hispanics, in both adult and pediatric populations (2–4). It is now the most common cause of nephrotic syndrome in adults in the U.S. Patients with FSGS may have hypertension and hematuria. Serologic studies, including complement levels, are typically within normal limits in both MCD and FSGS.

Pathologic Features

Light Microscopy

Minimal change disease shows normal glomeruli by light microscopy (Fig. 4.1). In FSGS, sclerosis involves some, but not all, glomeruli (focal), and the sclerosis affects a portion of, but not the entire, glomerular tuft (segmental) (Fig. 4.2) (1,5–7). Sclerosis is defined as increased matrix with obliteration of the capillary lumen. Uninvolved glomeruli in FSGS show no apparent lesions by light microscopy; FSGS may also entail hyalinosis, caused by insudation of plasma proteins, producing a smooth, glassy (hyaline) appearance (Fig. 4.3). Adhesions (synechiae) of the capillary tuft to Bowman's space are a very early sclerosing lesion.

Focal segmental glomerulosclerosis is diagnosed when even a single glomerulus shows segmental sclerosis. Therefore, samples must be adequate to detect these focal and segmental lesions. A biopsy with only 10 glomeruli has a 35% probability of missing a focal (10% involved) lesion, decreasing to 12% if 20 glomeruli are sampled (8). The juxtamedullary

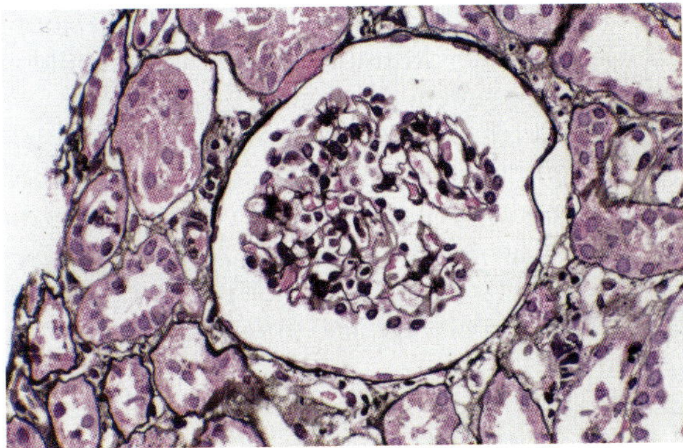

FIGURE 4.1. Normal glomeruli in minimal change disease (Jones silver stain).

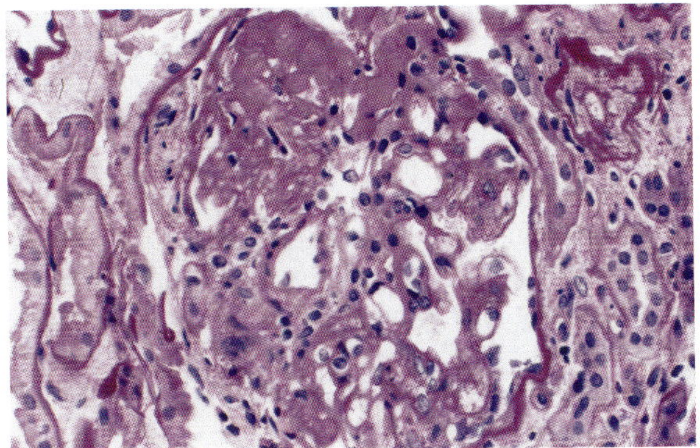

FIGURE 4.2. Glomerulosclerosis in focal and segmental pattern in focal segmental glomerulosclerosis, not otherwise specified (FSGS NOS) type [periodic acid-Schiff (PAS)].

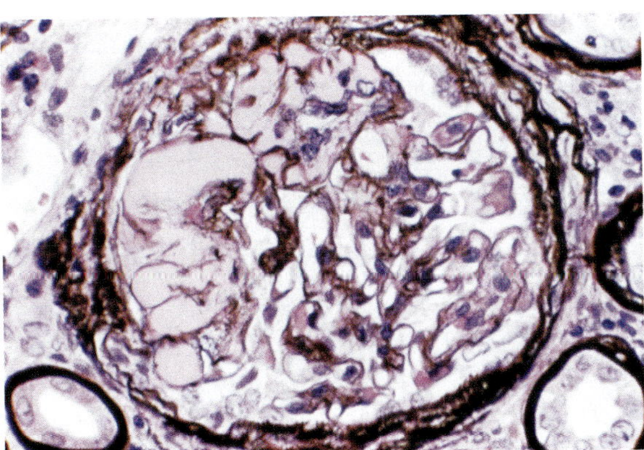

FIGURE 4.3. Extensive hyalinosis and sclerosis in FSGS NOS type (Jones silver stain).

region also should be included in the biopsy for optimal sampling, because that is where FSGS starts (5). Multiple step sections should also be examined to detect the focal segmental lesions.

Global glomerulosclerosis, in contrast to the segmental lesion, is not of special diagnostic significance in diagnosing FSGS. Globally sclerotic glomeruli may be normally seen at any age. In children, less than 1% global sclerosis is expected. The extent of global sclerosis increases with aging. Smith et al. (9) proffered the formula for normal percent of global sclerosis in adults of up to half the patient's age, minus 10, for example, up to 30% by age 80.

Morphologic variants of sclerosis appear to have differing prognosis (see below) (10,11). The most common type of FSGS, *FSGS not otherwise specified* (*NOS*), has no specific distinguishing features, and is characterized by segmental sclerosis, defined as increased matrix and obliteration of capillary lumina, often with hyalinosis in the absence of underlying immune complexes or other indicators of a secondary etiology by complete immunofluorescence/electron microscopy (IF/EM) evaluation; FSGS NOS is diagnosed by exclusion of specific subtypes as follows (Fig. 4.4): Collapsing variant of FSGS is characterized by collapse of the capillary loops and overlying podocyte proliferation, and has a particularly ominous prognosis (Fig. 4.5) (12,13). Even just one glomerulus with collapsing lesion is sufficient, we propose, to classify the process as collapsing variant FSGS. In the absence of collapsing lesions, the location of lesions, either peripheral or hilar, has significance as follows: The *glomerular tip lesion* is defined as sclerosis only affecting the tubular pole of the glomerulus, with adhesion of the tuft to the proximal tubule outlet (Fig. 4.6). There is often associated endocapillary hypercellularity and intracapillary foam cells (14–16). The

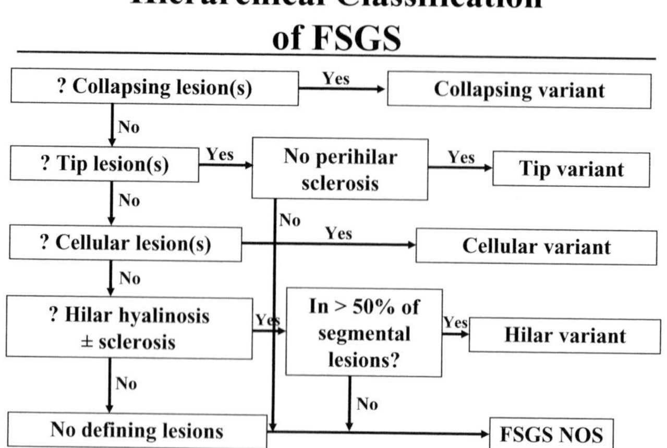

FIGURE 4.4. Hierarchical classification schema for FSGS variants.

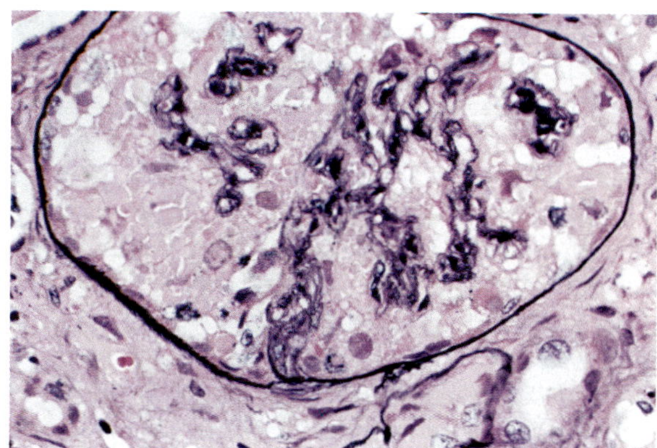

FIGURE 4.5. Collapse of glomerular tuft with overlying podocyte hyperplasia in collapsing type FSGS (Jones silver stain).

cellular variant of FSGS is characterized by segmental proliferative podocyte reaction associated with early sclerosis and/or endocapillary hypercellularity and often intracapillary foam cells (17). It does not, per definition, involve the tubular pole. Predominantly *hilar lesions*, that is, more than half of sclerotic glomeruli with sclerosis with associated hyaline at the hilar pole, in the absence of collapsing lesions, have been proposed to represent a response to reduced renal mass, and may also be associated with secondary FSGS seen with arterionephrosclerosis (10,11).

Vascular sclerosis may be prominent late in the course of FSGS and is proportional to glomerular sclerosis. Tubular atrophy is often accompanied

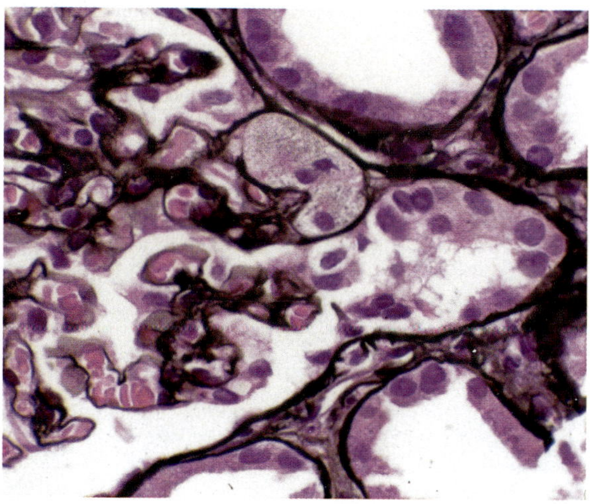

FIGURE 4.6. Adhesion and endocapillary foam cells at proximal tubular pole in tip variant of FSGS (Jones silver stain).

by interstitial fibrosis, proportional to the degree of scarring in the glomerulus. In HIV nephropathy and collapsing glomerulopathy, tubular lesions are disproportionally severe, with cystic dilation and a more prominent infiltrate (18).

The presence of acute interstitial nephritis (i.e., edema, interstitial infiltrate of lymphocytes, plasma cells, and often eosinophils), and apparent MCD glomerular lesion (i.e., complete foot process effacement, no light microscopic lesions) suggest a drug-induced hypersensitivity etiology, in particular nonsteroidal antiinflammatory drug (NSAID)-related injury.

Surrogate markers of unsampled FSGS have been sought to suspect FSGS even when sclerosed glomeruli are not detected. Abnormal glomerular enlargement (see below) appears to be an early indicator of the sclerotic process preceding overt sclerosis (19). Tubulointerstitial fibrosis in a young patient without sclerosis could also indicate possible unsampled FSGS.

Immunofluorescence Microscopy

There are no immune complex deposits in either MCD or FSGS. In FSGS, there may be nonspecific entrapment of immunoglobulin M (IgM) and C3 in sclerotic areas or areas where mesangial matrix is increased. IgM staining without deposits by EM does not appear to have specific diagnostic, prognostic, or etiologic significance (20).

Electron Microscopy

Electron microscopy shows foot process effacement, vacuolization, and microvillous transformation of epithelial cells in both MCD and FSGS. In MCD, foot process effacement is typically extensive (Fig. 4.7). Foot process

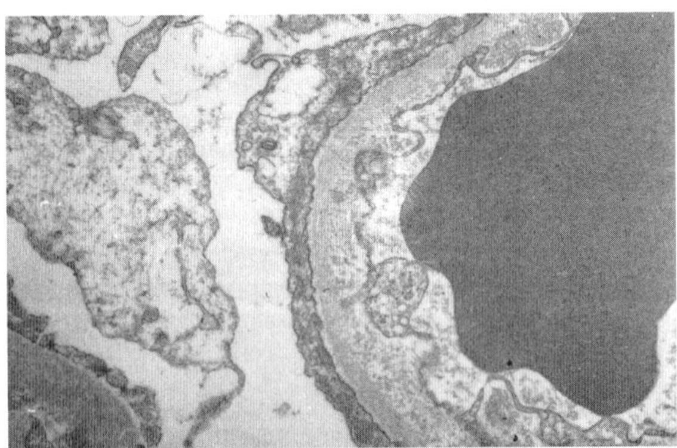

FIGURE 4.7. Extensive foot process effacement is present in minimal change disease, and also in FSGS. No immune complexes are present (electron microscopy).

effacement is often not complete in FSGS (20). However, the extent of foot process effacement does not allow precise distinction between the two disease processes. In secondary FSGS, foot process effacement is generally less than in idiopathic forms. In HIV-associated nephropathy (HIVAN), there are reticular aggregates in endothelial cell cytoplasm.

Etiology/Pathogenesis

The pathogenesis of MCD appears related to abnormal cytokines, which only affect glomerular permeability and do not promote sclerogenic mechanisms. Minimal change disease has been associated with drug-induced hypersensitivity reactions, bee stings, Hodgkin's disease, and other venom exposure, implicating immune dysfunction as an initiating factor.

Glomerular hypertrophy may be marker of FSGS. Glomerular enlargement precedes overt glomerulosclerosis in FSGS (19). Patients with abnormal glomerular growth on initial biopsies that did not show overt sclerotic lesions subsequently developed overt glomerulosclerosis, documented in later biopsies. A cutoff of glomerular area larger than 50% more than normal for age indicated increased risk for progression. Of note, glomeruli grow until approximately age 18 years, so age-matched controls must be used in the pediatric population. Since tissue processing methods may influence the size of structures in tissue, it is imperative that each laboratory determines normal ranges for this parameter.

Recurrence of FSGS in the transplant has also shed light on its pathogenesis (21). Most recurrences occur within the first months after transplantation, but recurrence may be immediate. Foot process effacement is present when proteinuria recurs and precedes the development of sclerosis, typically by weeks to months. A circulating factor has been identified in patients with recurrent FSGS, which induces increased ex vivo glomerular permeability, and also a mild increase in proteinuria when injected in rats (22). Plasmapheresis induced remission in some patients with recurrent FSGS, but more often relapse occurred when plasmapheresis was stopped.

Differentiation markers of podocytes, including the Wilms' tumor WT-1 protein, podocalyxin, and synaptopodin, are retained when proteinuria is caused by MCD or membranous glomerulonephritis (GN), but disappeared (or were decreased in the case of synaptopodin) in the collapsing variant of FSGS or HIV-associated nephropathy, with lesser changes in typical FSGS. These observations point to a dysregulated phenotype of the podocyte in the pathogenesis of the collapsing and HIV-associated forms of FSGS (23).

Studies of the molecular biology of the podocyte and identification of genes mutated in rare familial forms of nephrotic syndrome or FSGS, such as nephrin, α-actinin-4, and podocin, have given important new insights into mechanisms of progressive glomerulosclerosis. The gene mutated for congenital nephrotic syndrome, nephrin (*NPHS1*) is localized to chromosome region 19q13 (24). The common mutations in this syndrome are called *fin major* and *fin minor.* Nephrin localizes to the slit diaphragm over the podocyte and is tightly associated with CD2-associated protein (CD2AP) (25). Nephrin functions as a zona occludens–type junction protein, and along with CD2AP is thought to provide a crucial role in receptor patterning and cytoskeletal polarity. Recent data also show that nephrin has signal transduction functions. Surprisingly, some patients develop nephrotic syndrome after transplantation, if the original disease was due to *fin major* mutations, which leads to complete loss of nephrin. The mechanism for recurrent nephrotic syndrome is not determined. Mice engineered to be deficient in CD2AP develop congenital nephrotic syndrome, similar to congenital nephrotic syndrome of the Finnish type. Recently, mutations of CD2AP, predicted to cause loss of function, have been detected in two adult patients with proteinuria and presumed FSGS without a family history of the disease (26).

Additional important genes interacting with the nephrin-CD2AP complex have been identified in rare cases of familial FSGS (27,28). Autosomal dominant FSGS is caused by mutation in α-actinin-4 (ACTN4), also localized to chromosome 19q13 (29). Patients with the ACTN4 mutation progress to end stage by age 30, with rare recurrence in the transplant. The ACTN4 mutation is hypothesized to cause altered actin cytoskeleton interaction, causing FSGS through a gain-of-function mechanism, contrasting with the loss-of-function mechanism implicated for disease caused by the nephrin mutation. Mice with knock-in of mutated ACTN4 indeed develop FSGS, supporting this hypothesis (30). Podocin, another podocyte-specific gene (*NPHS2*) is mutated in autosomal recessive FSGS with an early onset in childhood with rapid progression to end stage (31). Podocin is an integral stomatin protein family member and interacts with the CD2AP-nephrin complex, indicating that podocin could serve in the structural organization of the slit diaphragm. Patients with sporadic FSGS and podocin mutation showed recurrence of FSGS after transplant at the same rate as the general FSGS population (32). Recently, an overlap in the *NPHS1*/*NPHS2* mutation spectrum has been detected, modifying the phenotype of congenital nephrotic syndrome of the Finnish type to congenital FSGS when mutations in both are inherited. These findings further point to key functional interrelationships between *NPHS1* and *NPHS2* (33). Acquired FSGS also may involve alteration in expression of some of these key podocyte genes. Indeed, some patients with nonfamilial forms of FSGS have been found to have podocin mutations. Importantly, patients with such podocin mutations are generally resistant to steroid therapy (34,35).

Additional observations underscore the importance of the interactions between the podocyte and the underlying basement membrane. Dystroglycan is an integral component of the GBM. Decreased dystroglycan staining was observed in patients with MCD (36). Dystroglycan expression was maintained in the nonsclerotic segments in FSGS, suggesting that MCD and FSGS are indeed different disease processes and not merely different stages of one disease.

Germline mutations of the WT-1 (Wilms' tumor) suppressor gene are found in Denys-Drash syndrome, a rare childhood disease with diffuse mesangial sclerosis, XY hermaphroditism, and a high risk of Wilms' tumor, with mutations usually of exon 9; and in Frasier syndrome, a disease with FSGS, XY hermaphroditism, and a high risk of gonadoblastoma, with mutations of intron 9 (37). Abnormal, lamellated basement membranes were observed in three patients with FSGS associated with Frasier syndrome, in whom studies for coexistent Alport syndrome were negative (38). Abnormal splice variants of WT-1 have rarely been associated with nonsyndromal cases of FSGS (39).

Clinicopathologic Correlations

Minimal change disease patients typically respond to corticosteroids, with excellent long-term prognosis. In contrast, FSGS usually results in progressive decline of GFR. The finding of *mesangial hypercellularity* was proposed to indicate a subtype of primary MCD with poorer prognosis and increased risk for development of FSGS. However, several series have failed to confirm a definite clinical correlation of this morphologic variant. Thus, diffuse mesangial hypercellularity does not appear to impart a specific prognostic significance, and is rather regarded as a manifestation of an earlier stage of disease.

The proposed morphologic variants of FSGS appear to have prognostic significance (Table 4.1) (10,11). Collapsing FSGS has a poor prognosis with rapid loss of renal function and virtually no responsiveness to corticosteroids alone (13). Series of patients with collapsing FSGS show

TABLE 4.1. Working classification of focal segmental glomerulosclerosis (FSGS)

Type	Key histologic feature	Possible prognostic implication
FSGS NOS	Segmental sclerosis	Typical course
Collapsing FSGS	Collapse of tuft, podocyte hyperplasia	Poor prognosis
Cellular FSGS	Endocapillary proliferation, often podocyte hyperplasia	?Early-stage lesion
Tip lesion	Sclerosis/adhesion at proximal tubule pole	?Better prognosis
Perihilar variant	Sclerosis and hyalinosis at vascular pole	?May reflect a secondary type of FSGS

NOS, not otherwise specified.

a strong preponderance of African Americans, and most patients were adults. The etiology has not yet been defined; however, a possible viral agent has been proposed. Evidence of parvovirus infection was increased in patients with collapsing glomerulopathy compared to controls, usual-type FSGS and HIVAN, suggesting an association (40). The drug pamidronate also has been linked to the development of collapsing glomerulopathy (41). Collapsing lesions also have been seen in the transplant, linked to cyclosporine toxicity.

Clinically, patients with the cellular variant of FSGS have an abrupt onset of nephrotic syndrome. These patients typically show transition to progressively less cellular, more sclerotic lesions, becoming indistinguishable clinically and morphologically from classical FSGS. This cellular lesion may be an early abnormality seen by light microscopy (LM) when FSGS recurs in the transplant. This morphologic appearance is postulated to represent an early, active lesion (10,11).

Tip lesions, that is, glomerulosclerosis involving the proximal tubular pole of the glomerulus, and not extending past the mid-region, were proposed to represent an early lesion with good prognosis, although later follow-up has revealed a less than benign prognosis in some patients (14,15). Review of autopsy cases of children with MCD who died of overwhelming infection showed rare tip lesions, suggesting that the lesion may not be disease specific (16). Tips lesions can occur at any age. Patients typically present with nephrotic syndrome. In one recent series, patients with the tip lesion variant of FSGS were compared to FSGS NOS and MCD patients. After treatment with steroids alone in most of the tip lesion patients, with added cytotoxic therapy in about a third, over half had achieved remission, whereas only one of 29 in whom follow-up was available progressed to ESRD (15). Thus, the tip variant appears to have a better prognosis than FSGS NOS and to be more similar to MCD.

Predominantly *hilar lesions*, with glomerulosclerosis located at the vascular pole with associated hyaline, have been proposed to represent a response to reduced renal mass, and may also be associated with secondary FSGS seen with arterionephrosclerosis.

Secondary and Other Variant Forms of Focal Segmental Glomerulosclerosis

C1q Nephropathy

C1q nephropathy is best considered as a variant of FSGS-like disease, and presents as nephrotic syndrome (42,43). These patients are generally adolescent African Americans, steroid resistant, and some of those with sclerosis have developed end-stage renal disease. The median time to end stage from biopsy was 81 months in one recent series of 19 patients. Clinical or morphological findings of lupus nephritis are absent [e.g., no reticular aggregates, no clinical evidence of systemic lupus erythematosus (SLE)].

By light microscopy, there may be no lesions or focal segmental sclerosis. Tubular atrophy and interstitial fibrosis are proportional to sclerosis.

Immunofluorescence microscopy may show staining with IgG, IgM, C3, but by definition has prominent C1q. The pattern is most often mesangial, but capillary loop staining may also be present.

Electron microscopy shows electron-dense mesangial deposits, with occasional extension to subendothelial areas. There are no reticular aggregates.

Tubular atrophy and interstitial fibrosis were the best correlates of renal insufficiency at biopsy and at follow-up. The prognosis of those without sclerosis at time of biopsies awaits further follow-up studies.

Secondary Focal Segmental Glomerulosclerosis

Many insults to the kidney may result in secondary FSGS, either as the sole manifestation of injury or superimposed on other renal disease manifestations (6,10). The lesion of FSGS may be seen in association with, for example, substantial loss of nephron mass, diabetes, obesity, HIV infection, or heroin abuse. Hilar-type sclerosis may often manifest with these secondary forms of FSGS (see above). Secondary sclerosis also occurs in the chronic stage of many immune complex or proliferative diseases. In some of these settings, the morphologic appearance of sclerosis can indicate the nature of the initial insult: obesity-associated FSGS shows mild mesangial expansion, GBM thickening, subtotal foot process effacement, and marked glomerulomegaly (44). The course is more indolent than for idiopathic FSGS with less frequent nephrotic syndrome. In FSGS secondary to reflux nephropathy, there is frequently prominent periglomerular fibrosis and thickening of Bowman's capsule and patchy interstitial scarring, in addition to the heterogeneous glomerulosclerosis. Focal segmental glomerulosclerosis associated with heroin use does not show pathognomonic features, although global glomerulosclerosis, epithelial cell changes, interstitial fibrosis, and tubular injury tend to be more prominent than in idiopathic cases of FSGS. In HIV-associated nephropathy, the tubules show severe injury, including cystic dilatation, out of proportion to the focal segmental glomerular scarring. Glomeruli show tuft collapse, and reticular aggregates are numerous in endothelial cells. Also, FSGS can develop in association with decreased renal mass, whether acquired or present at birth.

In summary, FSGS is a lesion with many manifestations and diverse mechanisms, including genetic, circulating factors, and environmental. Classification based on increasing understanding of these varying forms will likely lead to improved prognosis and, it is hoped, to treatments.

References

1. Southwest Pediatric Nephrology Study Group. A report: focal segmental glomerulosclerosis in children with idiopathic nephrotic syndrome. Kidney Int 27:442–449, 1985.
2. Haas M, Spargo B, Coventry S. Increasing incidence of focal-segmental glomerulosclerosis among adult nephropathies: a 20-year renal biopsy study. Am J Kidney Dis 26:740–750, 1995.
3. Braden GL, Mulhern JG, O'Shea MH, Nash SV, Ucci AA Jr, Germain MJ. Changing incidence of glomerular diseases in adults. Am J Kidney Dis 35:878–883, 2000.
4. Andreoli SP. Racial and ethnic differences in the incidence and progression of focal segmental glomerulosclerosis in children. Adv Ren Replace Ther 11:105–109, 2004.
5. Rich AR. A hitherto undescribed vulnerability of the juxta-medullary glomeruli in lipoid nephrosis. Bull Johns Hopkins Hosp 100:173–186, 1957.
6. D'Agati V. The many masks of focal segmental glomerulosclerosis. Kidney Int 46:1223–1241, 1994.
7. Fogo A, Glick AD, Horn SL, Horn RG. Is focal segmental glomerulosclerosis really focal? Distribution of lesions in adults and children. Kidney Int 47:1690–1696, 1995.
8. Corwin HL, Schwartz MM, Lewis EJ. The importance of sample size in the interpretation of the renal biopsy. Am J Nephrol 8:85–89, 1988.
9. Smith SM, Hoy WE, Cobb L. Low incidence of glomerulosclerosis in normal kidneys. Arch Pathol Lab Med 113:1253–1256, 1989.
10. D'Agati V. Pathologic classification of focal segmental glomerulosclerosis. Semin Nephrol 23:117–134, 2003.
11. D'Agati VD, Fogo AB, Bruijn JA, Jennette JC. Pathologic classification of focal segmental glomerulosclerosis: a working proposal. Am J Kidney Dis 43:368–382, 2004.
12. Detwiler RK, Falk RF, Hogan SL, Jennette JC. Collapsing glomerulopathy: a clinically and pathologically distinct Variant of focal segmental glomerulosclerosis. Kidney Int 45:1416–1424, 1994.
13. Valeri A, Barisoni L, Appel GB, Seigle R, D'Agati V. Idiopathic collapsing focal segmental glomerulosclerosis: a clinicopathologic study. Kidney Int 50:1734–1746, 1996.
14. Howie AJ, Brewer DB. Further studies on the glomerular tip lesion: early and late stages and life table analysis. J Pathol 147:245–255, 1985.
15. Stokes MB, Markowitz GS, Lin J, Valeri AM, D'Agati VD. Glomerular tip lesion: a distinct entity within the minimal change disease/focal segmental glomerulosclerosis spectrum. Kidney Int 65:1690–1702, 2004.
16. Haas M, Yousefzadeh N. Glomerular tip lesion in minimal change nephropathy: a study of autopsies before 1950. Am J Kidney Dis 39:1168–1175, 2002.
17. Chun MJ, Korbet SM, Schwartz MM, Lewis EJ. Focal segmental glomerulosclerosis in nephrotic adults: presentation, prognosis, and response to therapy of the histologic variants. J Am Soc Nephrol 15:2169–2177, 2004.
18. Cohen AH, Nast CC. HIV-associated nephropathy: a unique combined glomerular, tubular, and interstitial lesion. Mod Pathol 1:87–97, 1988.

19. Fogo A, Hawkins EP, Berry PL, et al. Glomerular hypertrophy in minimal change disease predicts subsequent progression to focal glomerular sclerosis. Kidney Int 38:115–123, 1990.
20. Fogo A, Ichikawa I. Focal segmental glomerulosclerosis—a view and review. Pediatr Nephrol 10:374–391, 1996.
21. Tejani A, Stablein DH. Recurrence of focal segmental glomerulosclerosis posttransplantation: a special report of the North American Pediatric Renal Transplant Cooperative Study. J Am Soc Nephrol 2 (12 suppl):S258–263, 1992.
22. Savin VJ, Sharma R, Sharma M, et al. Circulating factor associated with increased glomerular permeability to albumin in recurrent focal segmental glomerulosclerosis. N Engl J Med 334:878–883, 1996.
23. Barisoni L, Kriz W, Mundel P, D'Agati V. The dysregulated podocyte phenotype: a novel concept in the pathogenesis of collapsing idiopathic focal segmental glomerulosclerosis and HIV-associated nephropathy. J Am Soc Nephrol 10:51–56, 1999.
24. Ruotsalainen V, Ljungberg P, Wartiovaara J, et al. Nephrin is specifically located at the slit diaphragm of glomerular podocytes. Proc Natl Acad Sci USA 96:7962–7967, 1999.
25. Shih NY, Li J, Karpitskii V, et al. Congenital nephrotic syndrome in mice lacking CD2-associated protein. Science 286(5438):312–315, 1999.
26. Kim JM, Wu H, Green G, et al. CD2-associated protein haploinsufficiency is linked to glomerular disease susceptibility. Science 300(5623):1298–1300, 2003.
27. Gubler MC. Podocyte differentiation and hereditary proteinuria/nephrotic syndromes. J Am Soc Nephrol 14(suppl 1):S22–26, 2003.
28. Pollak MR. The genetic basis of FSGS and steroid-resistant nephrosis. Semin Nephrol 23:141–146, 2003.
29. Kaplan JM, Kim SH, North KN, et al. Mutations in ACTN4, encoding alpha-actinin-4, cause familial focal segmental glomerulosclerosis. Nat Genet 24:251–256, 2000.
30. Michaud JL, Lemieux LI, Dube M, Vanderhyden BC, Robertson SJ, Kennedy CR. Focal and segmental glomerulosclerosis in mice with podocyte-specific expression of mutant alpha-actinin-4. J Am Soc Nephrol 14:1200–1211, 2003.
31. Boute N, Gribouval O, Roselli S, et al. NPHS2, encoding the glomerular protein podocin, is mutated in autosomal recessive steroid-resistant nephrotic syndrome. Nat Genet 24:349–354, 2000.
32. Bertelli R, Ginevri F, Caridi G, et al. Recurrence of focal segmental glomerulosclerosis after renal transplantation in patients with mutations of podocin. Am J Kidney Dis 41:1314–1321, 2003.
33. Koziell A, Grech V, Hussain S, et al. Genotype/phenotype correlations of NPHS1 and NPHS2 mutations in nephrotic syndrome advocate a functional inter-relationship in glomerular filtration. Hum Mol Genet 11:379–388, 2002.
34. Karle SM, Uetz B, Ronner V, Glaeser L, Hildebrandt F, Fuchshuber A. Novel mutations in NPHS2 detected in both familial and sporadic steroid-resistant nephrotic syndrome. J Am Soc Nephrol 13:388–393, 2002.

35. Ruf RG, Lichtenberger A, Karle SM, et al. Arbeitsgemeinschaft Fur Padiatrische Nephrologie Study Group. Patients with mutations in NPHS2 (podocin) do not respond to standard steroid treatment of nephrotic syndrome. J Am Soc Nephrol 15:722–732, 2004.
36. Regele HM, Fillipovic E, Langer B, et al. Glomerular expression of dystroglycans is reduced in minimal change nephrosis but not in focal segmental glomerulosclerosis. J Am Soc Nephrol 11:403–412, 2000.
37. Auber F, Lortat-Jacob S, Sarnacki S, et al. Surgical management and genotype/phenotype correlations in WT1 gene-related diseases (Drash, Frasier syndromes). J Pediatr Surg 38:124–129, 2003.
38. Ito S, Hataya H, Ikeda M, et al. Alport syndrome-like basement membrane changes in Frasier syndrome: an electron microscopy study. Am J Kidney Dis 41:1110–1115, 2003.
39. Denamur E, Bocquet N, Baudouin V, et al. WT1 splice-site mutations are rarely associated with primary steroid-resistant focal and segmental glomerulosclerosis. Kidney Int 57:1868–1872, 2000.
40. Moudgil A, Nast CC, Bagga A, et al. Association of parvovirus B19 infection with idiopathic collapsing glomerulopathy. Kidney Int 59:2126–2133, 2001.
41. Markowitz GS, Appel GB, Fine PL, et al. Collapsing focal segmental glomerulosclerosis following treatment with high-dose pamidronate. J Am Soc Nephrol 12:1164–1172, 2001.
42. Jennette JC, Hipp CG. C1q nephropathy: a distinct pathologic entity usually causing nephrotic syndrome. Am J Kidney Dis 6:103–110, 1985.
43. Markowitz GS, Schwimmer JA, Stokes MB, et al. C1q nephropathy: a variant of focal segmental glomerulosclerosis. Kidney Int 64:1232–1240, 2003.
44. Kambham N, Markowitz GS, Valeri AM, Lin J, D'Agati VD. Obesity-related glomerulopathy: an emerging epidemic. Kidney Int 59:1498–1509, 2001.

Section III
Glomerular Disease with Nephritic Syndrome Presentations

5
Postinfectious Glomerulonephritis

Jan A. Bruijn

Introduction/Clinical Setting

Acute postinfectious glomerulonephritis is a kidney disease that follows after an infection. The most common and best understood form of acute postinfectious glomerulonephritis is poststreptococcal glomerulonephritis. Less is known about the other forms of postinfectious glomerulonephritis. In addition, there are glomerulonephritides that occur during persistent bacterial infections such as bacterial endocarditis, deep abscesses, and infected atrioventricular shunts in hydrocephalus (1).

A large number of bacterial, viral, and mycotic infections may be followed by acute glomerulonephritis. Especially after bacterial and viral infections, a proliferative form of glomerulonephritis occurs (2). In parasitic infections membranous or membranoproliferative forms are seen more often, with in general a worse prognosis. However, most cases of acute postinfectious glomerulonephritis are caused by group A streptococci and follow upper airway infections, such as pharyngitis or tonsillitis, by 14 to 21 days (3). Especially in warmer climates acute glomerulonephritis may also follow after skin infections. In recent decades the number of patients with poststreptococcal glomerulonephritis has decreased considerably in the United States and Europe. In the Western world, staphylococcus or gram-negative bacteria are now more often the cause of acute postinfectious glomerulonephritis than is streptococcus (4). In other parts of the world the incidence of poststreptococcal glomerulonephritis has remained high. In addition to the declining incidence, the number of biopsies with acute glomerulonephritis decreases because the clinician is less inclined to take a biopsy in a patient with classical or typical symptoms of acute postinfectious glomerulonephritis. The disease occurs especially in children between the ages of 2 and 12 years and young adults, and more often in men than in women (5–7). Clinically the disease is characterized by an acute nephritic syndrome (acute glomerulonephritis). The symptoms include an abrupt onset of macroscopic hematuria, oliguria, acute renal failure manifested by a sudden decrease in the glomerular filtration rate, and fluid retention manifested by edema and hypertension (3). Edema probably results from renal sodium retention caused by the sudden decrease in the glomerular filtration rate, rather than occurring as a consequence of hypoalbuminemia as in the nephrotic syndrome (6). Laboratory studies are directed at the urine sediment, proteinuria, renal function, and proving the immune response to streptococcal (antistreptolysin O, streptozyme) or viral antigens (3,8). Complement abnormalities include a large reduction in total serum hemolytic complement CH_{50} and C3 concentrations in many cases with normal C4, suggesting complement activation primarily via the alternative pathway (3).

Pathologic Findings

Light Microscopy

In acute glomerulonephritis usually all glomeruli are affected ("diffuse") and all to a similar extent ("global"). The glomerular capillaries are dilated and hypercellular, without necrosis. In addition to an increase of endothelial and mesangial cells, influx of inflammatory cells is present, especially neutrophilic granulocytes and monocytes (Fig. 5.1). Because of the large numbers of granulocytes the term *exudative glomerulonephritis* is used. Eosinophils and lymphocytes may occur, but they are usually scarce. The glomerular capillary walls are sometimes slightly thickened locally. In some biopsies using high magnification, small nodules may be seen on the epithelial side of the glomerular capillary walls, especially in the trichrome or toluidine-blue stains. These correspond to the subepithelial deposits ("humps") that are seen electron microscopically (see below). In severe cases extracapillary proliferation with formation of crescents and/or adhesions (synechiae) can be seen. In Bowman's space erythrocytes and some-

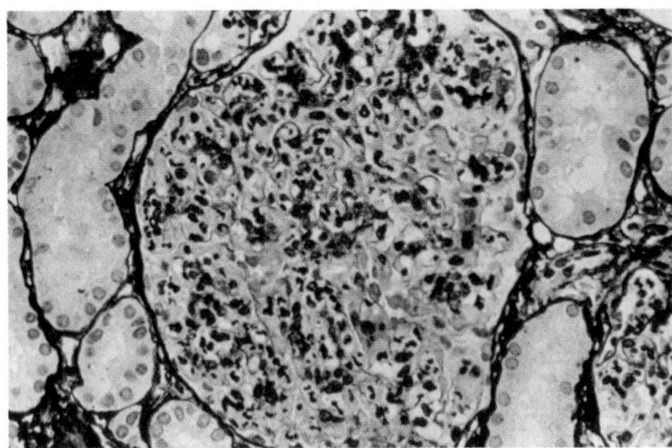

FIGURE 5.1. Diffusely hypercellular glomerulus in acute postinfectious glomerulonephritis with massive influx of neutrophilic polymorphonuclear granulocytes (Jones silver stain).

times granulocytes may be present. In renal biopsies taken a few weeks after the first clinical symptoms occurred, the picture is often more quiet. The number of granulocytes has decreased, the glomerular capillary walls have shrunk, the number of humps decreases, and the capillary walls are slender. In this stage diffuse mesangial hypercellularity may still be seen, and this can remain for several months. Evidence of resolving or largely healed postinfectious glomerulonephritis may be overlooked (9). This substantiates the contention that postinfectious glomerulonephritis occurs more frequently than is clinically appreciated (10).

Tubular changes are less prominent than glomerular alterations. When proteinuria occurs, reabsorption droplets can be seen in the proximal tubular epithelial cells. In the lumen of tubules protein cylinders, erythrocytes and sometimes granulocytes may be present. Tubular atrophy seldom occurs. The extent of interstitial damage varies, but is usually not extensive. Interstitial edema may be present with some mixed inflammatory infiltrate. Arteries and arterioles are usually unaffected.

Due to the combination of expansion of glomerular lobules, hypercellularity of the glomerular capillaries, and focal thickening of the capillary walls, postinfectious glomerulonephritis may be hard to distinguish from membranoproliferative glomerulonephritis light microscopically. Using immunofluorescence and electron microscopy a distinction between the two diseases can usually be made. However, a continuous, garland-type immunofluorescence pattern, although often considered typical for membranoproliferative glomerulonephritis, can also occur in postinfectious glomerulonephritis and is then related to a worse prognosis.

Immunofluorescence Microscopy

Immunofluorescence studies in biopsies taken during the first 2 to 3 weeks of the diseases most often show diffuse, irregular, coarse granular deposits of immunoglobulin G (IgG) and C3 along the glomerular capillary walls (Fig. 5.2). In large, confluent deposits the pattern may in places become continuous. In more than half of the cases IgM is also present, while IgA, IgE, and C1q are most often absent. Based on the distribution pattern of the immune complexes the morphology of postinfectious glomerulonephritis has been divided into several histologic subtypes, but these are not clearly related to clinical behavior or prognosis (11). Nasr and coworkers (12) described several cases of IgA-dominant acute poststaphylococcal glomerulonephritis complicating diabetic nephropathy.

Electron Microscopy

In acute glomerulonephritis, swelling of glomerular endothelial and mesangial cells is often seen electron microscopically. The glomerular basement membranes are usually of normal contour and thickness, although locally some thickening may occur. The glomerular basement membrane may also

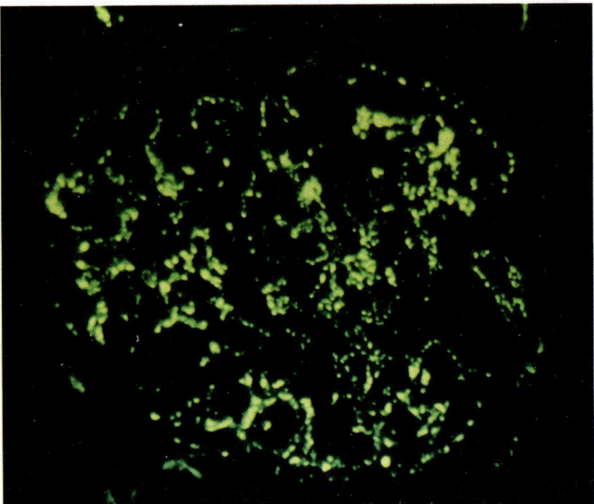

FIGURE 5.2. Immunofluorescence showing distribution of IgG in a "punctate" pattern in acute postinfectious glomerulonephritis.

contain electron-lucent areas, possibly representing "resolving" deposits. The glomerular endothelium is often damaged and denuded. The most consistent classic change, however, is the presence of glomerular subepithelial cone-shaped electron dense deposits, referred to as "humps." These are especially numerous during the first weeks of acute glomerulonephritis and their number decreases thereafter (Fig. 5.3). The humps are sometimes separated from the lamina densa by a lucent zone, which is in continuity with the lamina rara externa. Epithelial cell pedicles overlying the

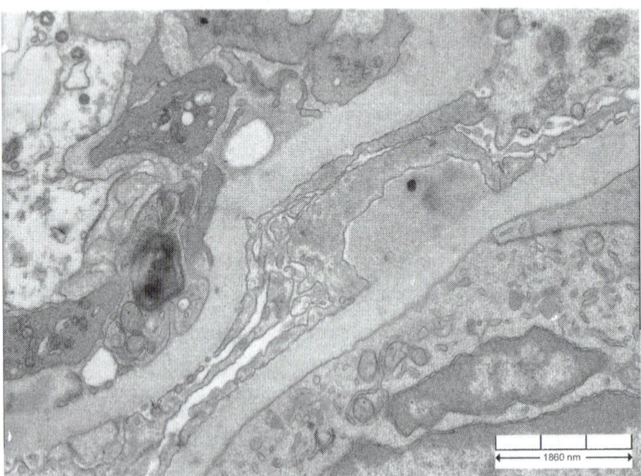

FIGURE 5.3. Electron microscopy showing large subepithelial electron dense deposits ("humps") and obliteration of visceral epithelial pedicles in acute postinfectious glomerulonephritis. Note absence of glomerular basement membrane (GBM) thickenings and spikes.

humps are often obliterated, with condensation of cytoplasmic microfilaments. In addition, some small irregular electron-dense deposits may be seen in the lamina densa, the mesangium, subendothelially, and sometimes along Bowman's capsule.

Etiology/Pathogenesis

Poststreptococcal nephritis is an immunologically mediated disease, in which both humoral and cellular immune mechanisms seem to play a role. In general, immune complexes deposited in the glomeruli could consist of either streptococcal antigen-antibody complexes or autologous antigen-antibody complexes. Over the years a large number of streptococcal antigenic fractions have been proposed as the putative target antigen, but only a few of these are still under active study (1). These include a protein fraction antigenically similar to streptokinase, and a cationic proteinase (13). Increasing evidence now points to an in situ antigen-antibody reactivity in poststreptococcal glomerulonephritis, as in a number of other glomerulonephritides (6,14,15). The cationic proteinase, due to its charge, is well able to pass the glomerular basement membrane and therefore should be able to induce subepithelial immune complex formation. The immune complexes induce further damage with the participation of the complement system and inflammatory cells as described in more detail in the chapters on membranous and lupus nephritides. The acute, nephritic, and endocapillary proliferative nature of poststreptococcal glomerulonephritis is probably related to the early phase of the disease, usually preceding the time of biopsy, during which immune complexes are present subendothelially. Subsequently, the immune complexes dissociate and transmigrate through the glomerular basement membrane to reassociate and form complexes subepithelially. The search for a genetic marker of the disease has been unsuccessful, although familial incidence of poststreptococcal glomerulonephritis is almost 40% (13).

Clinicopathologic Correlations

The prognosis of postinfectious glomerulonephritis with respect to renal function is in general good, with over 95% of patients recovering spontaneously with return to normal renal function within 3 to 4 weeks and with no long-term sequelae, even when renal failure is severe enough to need dialysis (3). The prognosis becomes worse when crescents are present, and in patients with severe proliferative glomerulonephritis the symptoms may progress to oliguria or anuria (5). The presence of proteinuria is prognostically a bad sign as well (16). The reported incidence of chronic renal insufficiency ranges from 0% to 20% (6). Novel molecular biologic techniques may allow more accurate determination of prognosis (17).

References

1. Silva FG. Acute postinfectious glomerulonephritis and glomerulonephritis complicating persistent bacterial infection. In: Jennette JC, Olson JL, Schwartz MM, Silva FG, eds. Heptinstall's Pathology of the Kidney, 5th ed. Philadelphia: Lippincott, 1998:389–453.
2. Sotsiou F. Postinfectious glomerulonephritis. Nephrol Dial Transplant 16(suppl 6):68–70, 2001.
3. Couser WG. Glomerulonephritis. Lancet 353:1509–1515, 1999.
4. Montseny JJ, Meyrier A, Kleinknecht D, Callard P. The current spectrum of infectious glomerulonephritis. Experience with 76 patients and review of the literature. Medicine (Baltimore) 74:63–73, 1995.
5. Kline Bolton W, Sturgill BC. Proliferative glomerulonephritis: postinfectious, noninfectious, and crescentic forms. In: Tisher CC, Brenner BM, eds. Renal Pathology. Philadelphia: Lippincott, 1989:156–195.
6. Hricik DE, Chung-Park M, Sedor JR. Glomerulonephritis. N Engl J Med 339:888–900, 1998.
7. Matsukura H, Ohtsuki A, Fuchizawa T, Miyawaki T. Acute poststreptococcal glomerulonephritis mimicking Henoch-Schönlein purpura. Clin Nephrol 59:64–65, 2003.
8. Mori Y, Yamashita H, Umeda Y, et al. Association of parvovirus B19 infection with acute glomerulonephritis in healthy adults: case report and review of the literature. Clin Nephrol 57:69–73, 2002.
9. Haas M. Incidental healed postinfectious glomerulonephritis: a study of 1012 renal biopsy specimens examined by electron microscopy. Hum Pathol 34:3–10, 2003.
10. Ruiz P, Soares M. Acute postinfectious glomerulonephritis: an immune response gone bad? Hum Pathol 34:1–2, 2003.
11. Edelstein CL, Bates WD. Subtypes of acute postinfectious glomerulonephritis: a clinico-pathological correlation. Clin Nephrol 38:311–317, 1992.
12. Nasr AH, Markowitz GS, Whelan JD, et al. IgA-dominant acute poststaphylococcal glomerulonephritis complicating diabetic nephropathy. Hum Pathol 34:1235–1241, 2003.
13. Rodriguez-Iturbe B. Glomerulonephritis associated with infection. In: Massry SG, Glassock RJ, eds. Textbook of Nephrology, 3rd ed. Baltimore: Williams & Wilkins, 1995:698–710.
14. Bruijn JA, Hoedemaeker PJ. Nephritogenic immune reactions involving native renal antigens. In: Massry SG, Glassock RJ, eds. Textbook of Nephrology, 3rd ed. Baltimore: Williams & Wilkins, 1995:627–631.
15. Bruijn JA, de Heer E, Hoedemaeker PJ. Immune mechanisms in injury to glomeruli and tubulo-interstitial tissue. In: Jones TC, ed. Monographs on Pathology of Laboratory Animals. Urinary System, 2nd ed. New York: Springer-Verlag, 1998:199–224.
16. Rodriguez-Iturbe B. Postinfectious glomerulonephritis. Am J Kidney Dis 35: xlvi–xlviii, 2000.
17. Eikmans M, Baelde JJ, de Heer E, Bruijn JA. RNA expression profiling as prognostic tool in renal patients: toward nephrogenomics. Kidney Int 62:1125–1135, 2002.

6
Immunoglobulin A Nephropathy and Henoch-Schönlein Purpura

J. Charles Jennette

Introduction/Clinical Setting

Immunoglobulin A (IgA) nephropathy was first described by the pathologist Jean Berger (1,2) and thus is sometimes called Berger's disease. Immunoglobulin A nephropathy is defined by the presence of IgA-dominant or co-dominant mesangial immunoglobulin deposits (Fig. 6.1) (3). Lupus glomerulonephritis, which may have IgA dominant or co-dominant deposits, is excluded from this diagnostic category. Immunoglobulin A nephropathy occurs as a primary (idiopathic) disease, as a component of Henoch-Schönlein purpura small-vessel vasculitis, secondary to liver disease (especially alcoholic cirrhosis), and associated with a variety of inflammatory diseases including ankylosing spondylitis, psoriasis, Reiter's disease, uveitis, enteritis (e.g., *Yersinia enterocolitica* infection), inflammatory bowel disease, celiac disease, dermatitis herpetiformis, and HIV infection (4–6).

Pathologic Findings

Light Microscopy

Immunoglobulin A nephropathy and Henoch-Schönlein purpura nephritis can have any of the histologic phenotypes of immune complex–mediated glomerulonephritis other than pure membranous glomerulopathy, including no lesion by light microscopy with immune deposits by immunohistology, mesangioproliferative glomerulonephritis with mesangial but no endocapillary hypercellularity (Figs. 6.2 and 6.3), focal or diffuse proliferative glomerulonephritis with endocapillary hypercellularity (with or without crescents) (Fig. 6.4), overt crescentic glomerulonephritis with 50% or more crescents, type I membranoproliferative (mesangiocapillary) glomerulonephritis (rare), and focal or diffuse sclerosing glomerulonephritis (7–10).

A variety of classification systems have been used to categorize the light microscopic phenotypes of IgA nephropathy, such as those proposed by

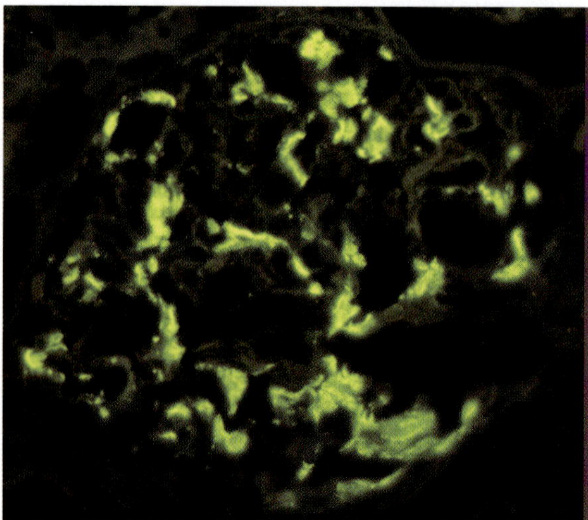

FIGURE 6.1. Immunofluorescence microscopy demonstrating glomerular mesangial staining for immunoglobulin A (IgA) in a patient with IgA nephropathy.

Kurt Lee et al (7) and by Mark Haas (8) (Table 6.1). Another approach is to use the same descriptive terminology that is in the World Health Organization (WHO) lupus classification system to categorize IgA nephropathy as well as other forms of immune complex glomerulonephritis. This system works as well for IgA nephropathy as it does for lupus, and also has the

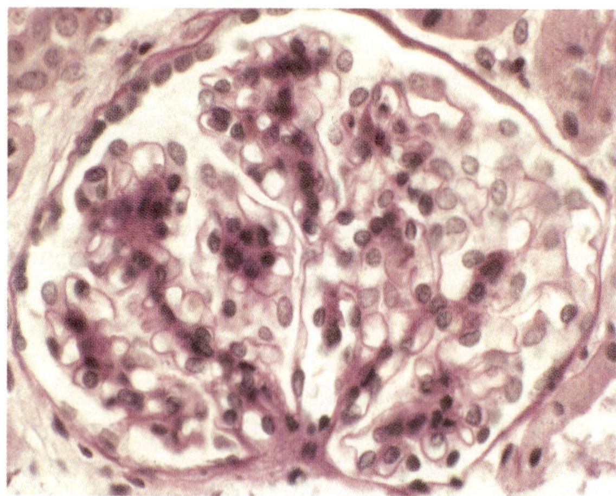

FIGURE 6.2. Glomerulus from a patient with IgA nephropathy showing mild segmental mesangial hypercellularity in the upper left quadrant of the glomerulus [periodic acid-Schiff (PAS) stain].

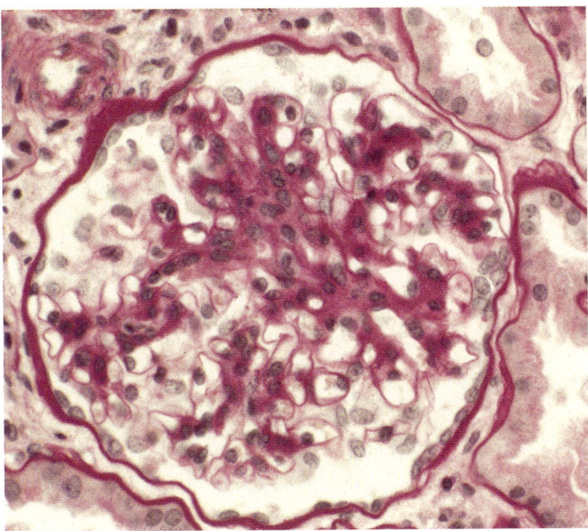

FIGURE 6.3. Glomerulus from a patient with IgA nephropathy showing moderate segmental mesangial hypercellularity and increased mesangial matrix in the upper portion of the tuft (PAS stain).

advantage of not requiring knowledge of multiple different classification systems.

In patients whose renal biopsy specimens are referred to the University of North Carolina for evaluation, crescents are observed in about a third of patients with IgA nephropathy and two thirds of patients with Henoch-

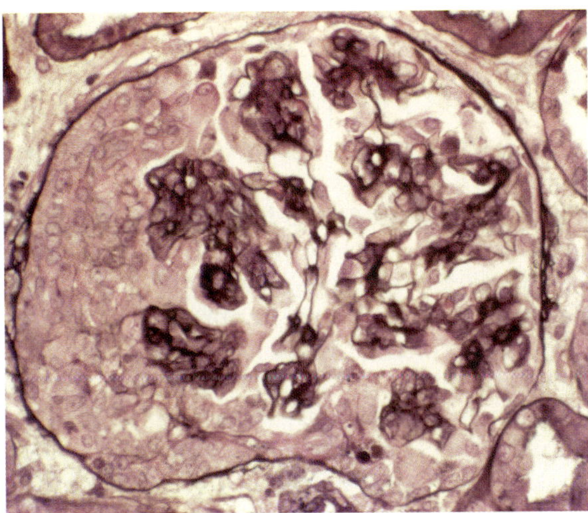

FIGURE 6.4. Glomerulus from a patient with Henoch-Schönlein purpura showing a proliferative glomerulonephritis with endocapillary hypercellularity adjacent to a cellular crescent on the right of the tuft (Jones silver stain).

TABLE 6.1. Three different approaches to the histologic classification of IgA nephropathy

Lee system	Haas system	WHO lupus terminology
I: Focal mesangioproliferative	I: Focal mesangioproliferative	I: Normal by light microscopy
II: Moderate focal proliferative	III: Focal proliferative	II: Focal mesangioproliferative
III: Mild diffuse proliferative	II: Focal sclerosing	III: Focal proliferative
IV: Moderate diffuse proliferative	IV: Diffuse proliferative	IIIC: Focal sclerosing
V: Severe diffuse proliferative	V: Chronic sclerosing	IV: Diffuse proliferative
		VI: Chronic sclerosing

Note: The Lee and Haas systems were specifically designed for IgA nephropathy, whereas the terminology for the World Health Organization (WHO) system was designed for lupus glomerulonephritis but can be used to describe the pathology of IgA nephropathy.

Schönlein purpura nephritis (11). However, overt crescentic glomerulonephritis with 50% of more of glomeruli with crescents is uncommon (<5% in IgA nephropathy and <10% in Henoch-Schönlein purpura nephritis). When substantial crescent formation is present, especially with conspicuous fibrinoid necrosis, the possibility of concurrent antineutrophil cytoplasmic antibody (ANCA) disease should be considered (12).

Between 5% and 10% of specimens with IgA nephropathy identified by immunohistology have focal segmental glomerular sclerosis as seen on light microscopy that is indistinguishable from idiopathic focal segmental glomerulosclerosis (8).

Immunofluorescence Microscopy

The sine qua non for a diagnosis of IgA nephropathy is immunohistologic detection of dominant or co-dominant staining for IgA in the glomerular mesangium (Fig. 6.1). A caveat to this is that the staining for IgA should at least be 1+ on a scale of 0 to 4+ or 0 to 3+. Trace amounts of IgA are not definitive evidence for IgA nephropathy. The IgA is predominantly IgA1 rather than IgA2. Capillary wall staining is observed in about a third of patients, and is more common in Henoch-Schönlein purpura nephritis (10). The mesangial immune deposits of IgA nephropathy stop abruptly at the glomerular hilum and are not observed along tubular basement membranes. Rare patients have IgA nephropathy concurrent with membranous glomerulopathy, and thus their specimens show granular capillary wall IgG staining and mesangial IgA dominant staining (13).

Staining for IgA essentially always is accompanied by staining for other immunoglobulins and complement components (3). Staining for IgG and IgM often is present, but at low intensity compared to IgA. A very distinctive feature of IgA nephropathy compared to other immune complex diseases is the predominance of staining for lambda over kappa light chains in many specimens. C3 staining is almost always present and usually relatively bright. However, staining for C1q is uncommon and when present is typically of low intensity. The presence of substantial C1q should raise the possibility of lupus nephritis with conspicuous IgA deposition. This suspicion would be supported further by finding endothelial tubuloreticular inclusions by electron microscopy and antinuclear antibodies serologically. As in other forms of glomerulonephritis, staining for fibrin is seen at sites of necrosis and crescent formation. Depending in part on what reagent antibody is used, the immune deposits occasionally stain for fibrin, especially in patients with Henoch-Schönlein purpura nephritis (10).

Electron Microscopy

The typical ultrastructural finding is immune complex–type electron-dense deposits in the mesangium (Figs. 6.5 and 6.6). Dense deposits most often are found immediately beneath the paramesangial glomerular basement membrane. The amount of deposits varies substantially, with occasional specimens having massive replacement of the matrix by the dense material (Fig. 6.6). Rare specimens that have well-defined IgA deposits by immunofluorescence microscopy do not have detectable mesangial dense deposits, which does not rule out a diagnosis of IgA nephropathy because the

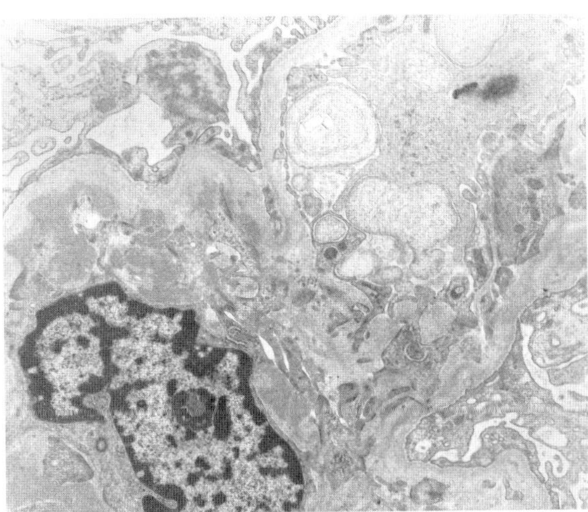

FIGURE 6.5. Electron micrograph of a glomerulus from a patient with IgA nephropathy showing a moderate amount of electron-dense deposits within the mesangium. The mesangium is on the left of the image and a portion of the capillary loop is on the right.

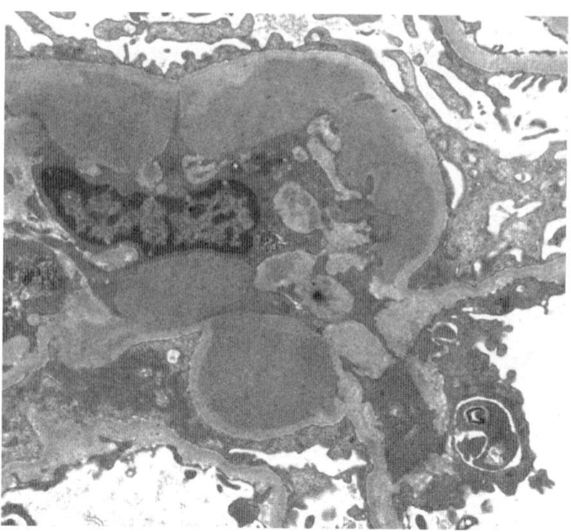

FIGURE 6.6. Electron micrograph of a glomerulus from a patient with IgA nephropathy showing massive electron-dense deposits within the mesangium. The mesangium is on the left of the image and a portion of the capillary loop is on the right.

immunohistology is the defining feature. Capillary wall subepithelial, subendothelial, and intramembranous deposits are identified in approximately a quarter to a third of specimens with IgA nephropathy (3), and are more frequent in patients with Henoch-Schönlein purpura nephritis (10). Capillary wall deposits are least frequent in histologically mild disease and most frequent in histologically severe disease, especially when crescents are present.

Focal areas of glomerular basement membrane thinning are observed in many specimens with IgA nephropathy (14). This structural abnormality may contribute to the hematuria. Focal or diffuse podocyte foot process effacement often is present, especially in patients with nephrotic range proteinuria. Foot process effacement is particularly prominent in patients who have the syndrome of histologically mild IgA nephropathy with minimal change glomerulopathy-like features clinically (15). Mesangial matrix expansion and mesangial hypercellularity parallel the mesangial changes seen by light microscopy.

Etiology/Pathogenesis

Immunoglobulin A nephropathy probably can result from multiple different etiologies and pathogenic processes, such as (1) abnormal structure and function of IgA molecules, (2) reduced clearance of circulating IgA complexes, (3) increased affinity for or reduced clearance of IgA deposits from the glomerular mesangium, (4) excessive IgA antibody production in response to mucosal antigen exposure, (5) excessive mucosal exposure to antigens, (6) increased permeability of mucosa to antigen, or (7) combinations of these factors.

Some secondary forms of IgA nephropathy appear to be caused by either decreased clearance of IgA from the circulation (e.g., reduced hepatic clearance caused by cirrhosis) or increased entry of IgA complexes into the circulation (e.g., caused by increased synthesis and greater access to the circulation in inflammatory bowel disease).

However, an important pathogenic mechanism in many patients with IgA nephropathy and Henoch-Schönlein purpura nephritis appears to derive from abnormally reduced galactosylation of the O-linked glycans in the hinge region of IgA1 molecules (6,16). This abnormality could result in mesangial IgA deposition by a variety of mechanisms including reduced clearance from the circulation because of lack of receptor engagement by the abnormal IgA, increased aggregation of IgA in the circulation resulting in mesangial trapping, development of immune complex–forming autoantibodies directed against the abnormal IgA, increased affinity of the abnormal IgA for mesangial matrix, or combinations of these processes.

Clinicopathologic Correlations

Immunoglobulin A nephropathy is said to be the most common form of glomerulonephritis in the world (4). The prevalence of IgA nephropathy varies among different racial groups, with the highest prevalence among Asians and Native Americans, intermediate prevalence among Caucasians, and lowest prevalence among individuals of African descent (4). Immunoglobulin A nephropathy and Henoch-Schönlein purpura nephritis are twice as common in males as females. On average, Henoch-Schönlein purpura nephritis occurs at an earlier age than IgA nephropathy (9). The onset and diagnosis of IgA nephropathy usually is in late childhood or early adulthood, whereas Henoch-Schönlein purpura usually occurs in children younger than 10 years of age. Immunoglobulin A nephropathy can manifest any of the signs and symptoms caused by glomerular disease. The most common initial manifestations are asymptomatic microscopic hematuria or intermittent gross hematuria or both. Approximately 10% of patients present with nephrotic syndrome and approximately 10% have renal failure at initial presentation. Rare patients present with rapidly progressive glomerulonephritis (17) or advanced chronic renal failure. Approximately 10% to 15% of patients reach end-stage renal disease within 10 years of diagnosis, and approximately 25% to 35% within 20 years (5,10). Immunoglobulin A nephropathy has a recurrence rate of greater than 50% in renal transplants. Recurrent IgA nephropathy causes some graft dysfunction in approximately 15% of patients after 5 years and graft loss in approximately 5% after 5 years (18).

The glomerulonephritis of Henoch-Schönlein purpura is not pathologically distinguishable from IgA nephropathy, although, as noted earlier, on average, Henoch-Schönlein purpura nephritis tends to be more severe with a higher frequency of crescent formation (10). In addition to nephritis, common clinical manifestations of Henoch-Schönlein purpura include arthralgias, purpura caused by leukocytoclastic angiitis of dermal capillaries, and abdominal pain caused by involvement of small vessels in the gut and other abdominal viscera (19). The presence of IgA deposits without vasculitis in systemic vessels is not adequate for a diagnosis of Henoch-Schönlein purpura because some patients with IgA nephropathy have no evidence for systemic vasculitis IgA deposits in extrarenal vessels, such as dermal venules. Patients with Henoch-Schönlein purpura usually have only one episode of purpura that resolves completely. Persistent and progressive nephritis is the most important long-term complication and results in end-stage disease in 5% to 20% of patients after 20 years (9).

The outcome of IgA nephropathy cannot be accurately predicted on the basis of clinical or pathologic features; however, as with other glomerular diseases, there are trends toward worse outcomes with more severe renal insufficiency at presentation, greater proteinuria, extensive crescent formation, or more extensive glomerular or tubulointerstitial scarring (6).

The treatment for IgA nephropathy remains controversial (4–6). There is general agreement that angiotensin-converting enzyme inhibitors are beneficial. Fish oil supplements with high concentrations of omega-3 fatty acids have been advocated by some investigators, but the evidence of their benefit is not conclusive. As with other forms of glomerulonephritis, corticosteroid treatment may be helpful, especially when there is substantial active glomerular inflammation or the syndrome with concurrent minimal change-like glomerulopathy. Treatment with cytotoxic agents generally has been reserved for patients with severe crescentic IgA nephropathy or Henoch-Schönlein purpura nephritis (17). It is hoped that the emerging knowledge of the pathogenesis of IgA nephropathy and Henoch-Schönlein purpura will lead to more effective treatment strategies.

References

1. Berger J, Hinglais N. Les depots intercapillaires d'IgA-IgG. J Urol 74:694–695,1968.
2. Berger J. IgA glomerular deposits in renal disease. Transplant Proc 1:939–944, 1969.
3. Jennette JC. The immunohistology of IgA nephropathy. Am J Kidney Dis 12:348–352, 1988.
4. Galla JH. IgA nephropathy. Kidney Int 47:377–387, 1995.
5. Donadio JV, Grande JP. Immunoglobulin A nephropathy: a clinical perspective. J Am Soc Nephrol 8:1324–1332, 1997.

6. Barratt J, Feehally J. IgA nephropathy. J Am Soc Nephrol 16:2088–2097, 2005.
7. Lee SMK, Rao VM, Franklin WA, et al. IgA nephropathy: morphologic predictors of progressive renal disease. Hum Pathol 13:314–322, 1982.
8. Haas M. Histologic subclassification of IgA nephropathy: a clinicopathologic study of 244 cases. Am J Kidney Dis 29:829–842, 1997.
9. Rai A, Nast C, Adler S. Henoch-Schoenlein purpura nephritis. J Am Soc Nephrol 10:2637–2644, 1999.
10. Davin JC, Ten Berge IJ, Weening JJ. What is the difference between IgA nephropathy and Henoch-Schoenlein purpura nephritis? Kidney Int 59:823–834, 2001.
11. Jennette JC. Rapidly progressive and crescentic glomerulonephritis. Kidney Int 63:1164–1172, 2003.
12. Haas M, Jafri J, Bartosh SM, Karp SL, Adler SG, Meehan SM. ANCA-associated crescentic glomerulonephritis with mesangial IgA deposits. Am J Kidney Dis 36:709–718, 2000.
13. Jennette JC, Newman WJ, Diaz-Buxo JA. Overlapping IgA and membranous nephropathy. Am J Clin Pathol 88:74–78, 1987.
14. Cosio FG, Falkenhain ME, Sedmak DD. Association of thin glomerular basement membrane with other glomerulopathies. Kidney Int 46:471–474, 1994.
15. Clive DM, Galvanek EG, Silva FG. Mesangial immunoglobulin A deposits in minimal change nephrotic syndrome: a report of an older patient and review of the literature. Am J Nephrol 10:31–36, 1990.
16. Hiki Y, Kokubo T, Iwase H, et al. Underglycosylation of IgA1 hinge plays a certain role for its glomerular deposition in IgA nephropathy. J Am Soc Nephrol 10:760–769, 1999.
17. Tumlin JA, Hennigar RA. Clinical presentation, natural history, and treatment of crescentic proliferative IgA nephropathy. Semin Nephrol 24:256–268, 2004.
18. Floege J. Recurrent IgA nephropathy after renal transplantation. Semin Nephrol 24:287–291, 2004.
19. Jennette JC, Falk RJ. Small vessel vasculitis. N Engl J Med 337:1512–1523, 1997.

7
Thin Basement Membranes and Alport's Syndrome

Agnes B. Fogo

Introduction/Clinical Setting

Classical Alport's syndrome is an X-linked disease and is the most common form of Alport's syndrome (90% of patients), with an overall incidence of Alport's syndrome in the United States of 1:5000 to 1:10,000 (1–4). Patients show hematuria in childhood with progressive hearing loss in one third, and ocular defects and progression to renal failure in 30% to 40% by early adulthood. Anterior lenticonus is the most common eye defect.

Alport syndrome is due to mutations of collagen type IV (3–6). Collagen type IV is made up of heterotrimers of alpha chains. These six alpha chains are encoded by genes arranged in pairs on three different chromosomes: *COL4A1* and *COL4A2* are on chromosome 13; *COL4A3* and *COL4A4* are on chromosome 2; and *COL4A5* and *COL4A6* are on the X chromosome. The mutation in the classic form of Alport's occurs in the α5 (IV) collagen chain (*COL4A5*). The autosomal recessive form accounts for most of the remaining patients, and is due to mutations in both alleles of α3 or α4 type IV collagen genes (*COL4A3* or *COL4A4*). Rare cases of autosomal dominant Alport's due to heterozygous mutations in *COL4A3* or *COL4A4* also occur, with a highly variable clinical course and reduced penetrance (7). Alport's syndrome and coexisting diffuse leiomyomatosis is linked to large gene deletions that span the adjacent 5′ ends of the adjacent *COL4A5* and *COL4A6* genes (5).

Pathologic Findings

Light Microscopy

There are no significant light microscopic abnormalities early in the disease (1). At later stages, glomerulosclerosis, interstitial fibrosis, and prominent interstitial foam cells, nonspecific and just indicative of proteinuria, are typical. Glomeruli show varying stages of matrix expansion and sclerosis.

Immunofluorescence Microscopy

Standard immunofluorescence (IF) may show nonspecific trapping of immunoglobulin M (IgM) in the mesangium. Special IF studies for subtypes of type IV collagen on either skin or renal biopsy may be helpful in distinguishing between causes of thin glomerular basement membrane (GBM), which may be the only lesion in early Alport, the carrier state for Alport, or so-called benign familial hematuria (see below) (3,5,8–11).

In kidney biopsies, about 70% to 80% of males with X-linked Alport's lack staining of the GBM, distal tubular basement membrane, and Bowman's capsule for α3, α4, or α5 (IV) chains, and Bowman's capsule and distal tubular basement membrane (TBM) also show lack of α6 (IV) (3,10,11). In autosomal recessive Alport's, where α3 or α4 is mutated, the kidney GBMs usually show no expression of α3, α4, or α5, again because there is an inability to form the normal α3, α4, or α5 type IV collagen heterotrimer of the GBM. In these autosomal recessive cases, in contrast to X-linked cases, α5 and α6 remain strongly expressed in Bowman's capsule, distal tubular basement membrane, and skin, because the $\alpha(1)_2 2/(5)_2 6$ heterotrimers can still be assembled in these patients. Female heterozygotes for X-linked Alport's syndrome frequently show mosaic staining of GBM and distal TBM for α3, α4, and α5 (IV) chains, and skin mosaic staining for α5 (IV). Patients with autosomal dominant Alport's have not been studied immunohistochemically.

Of note, some cases with Alport's syndrome clinically and by renal biopsy showed apparent normal α5 type IV immunostaining pattern. About 20% of male classic Alport patients and affected homozygous autosomal recessive Alport patients show faint or even normal staining of the skin or GBM for α3 and α5 (3). This is postulated to reflect a mutation that results in protein, that albeit abnormal, still expresses the epitope recognized by the available antibodies. Thus, the absence of α5 type IV in the skin biopsy is helpful in indicating a basement membrane abnormality, but an apparent normal staining pattern in either skin or kidney does not definitively rule out Alport's syndrome (10,11). The possible continuum of Alport's syndrome with some cases of apparent benign familial hematuria with thin basement membranes further complicates interpretation of staining patterns (see below).

Electron Microscopy

The diagnostic lesion consists of irregular thinned and thickened areas of the GBM with splitting and irregular multilaminated appearance of the lamina densa, so-called basket weaving (Fig. 7.1) (2). In between these lamina, granular, mottled material is present. In children with classic Alport's, the GBM may show only thinning rather than thickening. Female carriers of the *COL4A5* mutation also show only thin basement mem-

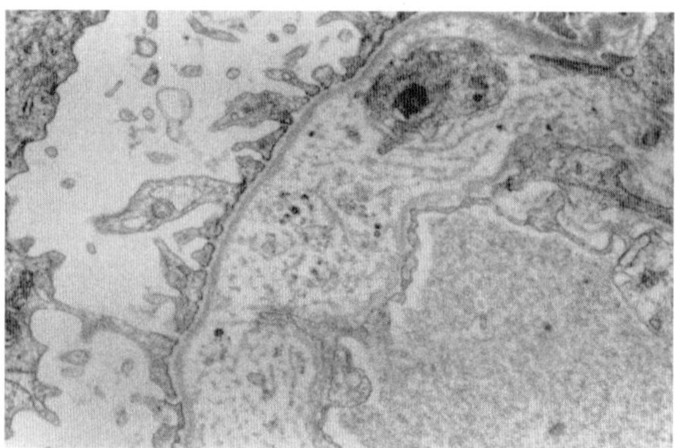

FIGURE 7.1. The glomerular basement membrane (GBM) is thickened with "basket-weaving" appearance, diagnostic of Alport's syndrome (electron microscopy).

branes, as do carriers of the autosomal recessive form of Alport's. The GBM thickness normally increases with age (12–14). Normal thickness in adults in one series was 373 ± 42 nm in men versus 326 ± 45 nm in women. Glomerular basement thickness <250 nm has been used as a cutoff for diagnosis in many series. In children, the diagnosis of thin basement membranes must be made with caution, establishing normal age-matched controls within each laboratory. In our laboratory, we found a range of GBM thickness in normal children from approximately 110 nm at age 1 year to 222 ± 14 nm in 7-year-olds.

Etiology/Pathogenesis

Alport's syndrome results from the inability to form normal type IV collagen heterotrimers. When α5 (or α3 or α4) is mutated, there is an inability to form the normal heterotrimers of the GBM. The organs involved in Alport's syndrome reflect sites where these type IV collagen chains are normally expressed and are essential for function, namely the kidney, eye, and ear. In the kidney, heterotrimers of α3, α4, and α5 type IV collagen are expressed in the GBM, whereas $\alpha(1)_2 2/(5)_2 6$ heterotrimers are expressed in Bowman's capsule and in some tubular basement membranes (5). At birth, $\alpha(1)_2 2$ heterotrimers are normally present in the immature glomerulus in the GBM, with gradual shift to the mature expression pattern. In the normal adult $\alpha(1)_2 2$ remains expressed in the mesangium and also in Bowman's capsule. The switch to normal adult α3, α4, α5 heterotrimers in the GBM cannot occur in Alport due to mutation in one of these chains. The mechanism(s) of progressive renal scarring in Alport's syndrome are unknown. In a report of seven patients with Alport's syndrome, decreased proteinuria occurred in response to angiotensin-converting enzyme inhibitor (ACEI), and, after an initial decrease of the glomerular filtration rate (GFR), renal function increased toward the starting levels by 24 months (15).

Each Alport kindred reported thus far has presented its own unique mutation. More than 300 mutations in the *COL4A5* gene have been identified (4). The rate of progression to end stage and deafness in hemizygous affected males are mutation dependent. Large deletions, nonsense mutations, or mutations that changed the reading frame were associated with 90% risk of end-stage renal disease before age 30 in affected males with X-linked Alport's, with only 50% risk for patients with missense and 70% risk for those with splice site mutations. Risk for hearing loss before age 30 was 60% in patients with missense mutations, versus 90% risk for all other mutations (16). Ultrastructural features do not strictly correlate with type of mutation, in that some patients with major gene rearrangements had no significant lesions, and varying ultrastructural abnormalities were present even within the same kindred (2).

Transplantation in patients with Alport's syndrome has shed additional light on the molecular basis for this disease. Some patients with Alport's receiving kidney transplants, probably around 5% to 10%, develop antibodies to the normal GBM in the transplant. Occurrence of this posttransplant anti-GBM disease appears more frequent in patients with more extensive deletion of the α5 type IV gene (5).

Thin Basement Membranes

Introduction/Clinical Setting

This basement membrane abnormality has also been described as "benign familial hematuria," and shows autosomal dominant or recessive inheritance (12–14). The clinical manifestation is that of chronic hematuria, either macroscopic or microscopic, intermittent or continuous. This lesion is common, and is present in 20% to 25% of patients biopsied for persistent isolated hematuria in some series, and may occur in more than 1% of the general population (17). The lesion may also coexist with other glomerular disease, commonly diabetic nephropathy or IgA nephropathy (18,19). Occasionally patients with thin basement membranes have nephrotic range proteinuria, with five of eight such cases in one series showing additional focal segmental glomerulosclerosis (FSGS) lesions (20).

Pathologic Findings

Light Microscopy

The light microscopic appearance is unremarkable.

Immunofluorescence Microscopy

Standard IF is negative. Special IF studies for type IV collagen molecules (see above) may identify some of the patients with thin basement membrane lesions as carriers or early-stage Alport (21).

Electron Microscopy

Diffuse, greater than 50%, thinning of GBM indicates possible thin basement membrane lesion, while small segmental areas of thinning are nonspecific (Fig. 7.2). The diagnosis of thin basement membranes is based on morphometric measurements from electron microscopic examination (see above). As mentioned above, thin basement membranes (without lamellation) may also be an early or only manifestation in some kindreds with Alport's syndrome. Thus, the presence of thin basement membranes cannot per se be taken to categorically indicate a benign prognosis.

Etiology/Pathogenesis

Numerous studies indicate that autosomal recessive Alport's syndrome and benign familial hematuria/thin basement membrane disease may represent a spectrum of severe to mild or carrier forms, respectively, of varying molecular defects in the same genes. Linkage of hematuria to mutations in either α4 type IV or α3 type IV has been documented in about 40% of kindreds with apparent thin basement membrane nephropathy clinically (17,21–23). In remaining kindreds without apparent linkage, de novo mutations or incomplete penetrance of the hematuria phenotype is proposed to occur. In one study of patients with thin basement membranes, there was

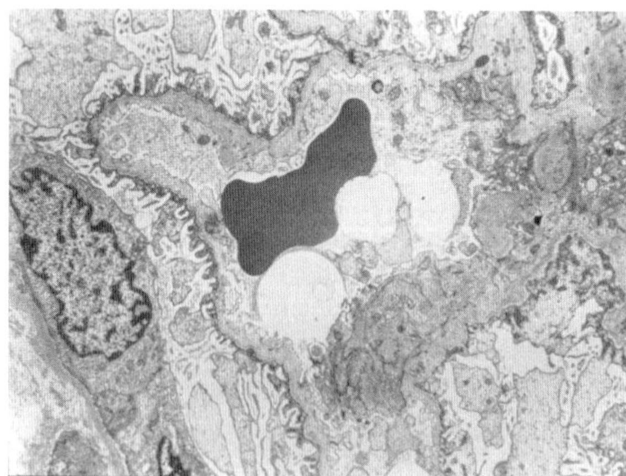

FIGURE 7.2. The GBM is diffusely thin in this adult with hematuria. Family history and immunostaining were consistent with thin basement membrane lesion of benign familial hematuria (electron microscopy).

increased global sclerosis, with later development of hypertension and renal insufficiency in the patients, and also in some relatives (24). However, these patients were not defined molecularly, and were presumed to not have Alport's syndrome based on absence of hearing or eye abnormalities.

References

1. Churg J, Sherman RL. Pathologic characteristics of hereditary nephritis. Arch Pathol 95:374, 1973.
2. Mazzucco G, Barsotti P, Muda AO, et al. Ultrastructural and immunohistochemical findings in Alport's syndrome: a study of 208 patients from 97 Italian families with particular emphasis on COL4A5 gene mutation correlations. J Am Soc Nephrol 9:1023–1031, 1998.
3. Pirson Y. Making the diagnosis of Alport's syndrome. Kidney Int 56:760–775, 1999.
4. Kashtan CE. Familial hematuria due to type IV collagen mutations: Alport syndrome and thin basement membrane nephropathy. Curr Opin Pediatr 16:177–181, 2004.
5. Hudson BG, Kalluri R, Tryggvason K. Pathology of glomerular basement membrane nephropathy. Curr Opin Nephrol Hypertens 3:334–339, 1994.
6. Longo I, Porcedda P, Mari F, et al. COL4A3/COL4A4 mutations: from familial hematuria to autosomal-dominant or recessive Alport syndrome. Kidney Int 61:1947–1956, 2002.
7. Pescucci C, Mari F, Longo I, et al. Autosomal-dominant Alport syndrome: natural history of a disease due to COL4A3 or COL4A4 gene. Kidney Int 65:1598–1603, 2004.
8. Nakanishi K, Yoshikawa N, Iijima K, et al. Immunohistochemical study of alpha 1–5 chains of type IV collagen in hereditary nephritis. Kidney Int 46:1413–1421, 1994.
9. Yoshioka K, Hino S, Takemura T, et al. Type IV collagen α5 chain. Normal distribution and abnormalities in X-linked Alport syndrome revealed by monoclonal antibody. Am J Pathol 144:986–996, 1994.
10. Kashtan CE. Alport syndrome: is diagnosis only skin-deep? Kidney Int 55:1575–1576, 1999.
11. Kashtan CE. Alport syndromes: phenotypic heterogeneity of progressive hereditary nephritis. Pediatr Nephrol 14:502–512, 2000.
12. Yoshiokawa N, Matsuyama S, Iijima K, Maehara K, Okada S, Matsuo T. Benign familial hematuria. Arch Pathol Lab Med 112:794–797, 1988.
13. Tiebosch ATMG, Frederik PM, van Breda Vriesman PJC, et al. Thin-basement-membrane nephropathy in adults with persistent hematuria. N Engl J Med 320:14–18, 1989.
14. Hisano S, Kwano M, Hatae K, et al. Asymptomatic isolated microhaematuria: natural history of 136 children. Pediatr Nephrol 5:578–581, 1991.
15. Proesmans W, Knockaert H, Trouet D. Enalapril in paediatric patients with Alport syndrome: 2 years' experience. Eur J Pediatr 159:430–433, 2000.
16. Jais JP, Knebelmann B, Giatras I, et al. X-linked Alport syndrome: natural history in 195 families and genotype-phenotype correlations in males. J Am Soc Nephrol 11:649–657, 2000.

17. Savige J, Rana K, Tonna S, Buzza M, Dagher H, Wang YY. Thin basement membrane nephropathy. Kidney Int 64:1169–1178, 2003.
18. Matsumae T, Fukusaki M, Sakata N, Takebayashi S, Naito S. Thin glomerular basement membrane in diabetic patients with urinary abnormalities. Clin Nephrol 42:221–226, 1994.
19. Cosio FG, Falkenhain ME, Sedmak DD. Association of thin glomerular basement membrane with other glomerulopathies. Kidney Int 46:471–474, 1994.
20. Nogueira M, Cartwright J Jr, Horn K, et al. Thin basement membrane disease with heavy proteinuria or nephrotic syndrome at presentation. Am J Kidney Dis 35:E15, 2000.
21. Liapis H, Gokden N, Hmiel P, Miner JH. Histopathology, ultrastructure, and clinical phenotypes in thin glomerular basement membrane disease variants. Hum Pathol 33:836–845, 2002.
22. Lemmink HH, Nillesen WN, Mochizuki T, et al. Benign familial hematuria due to mutation of the type IV collagen α4 gene. J Clin Invest 98:1114–1118, 1996.
23. Buzza M, Wang YY, Dagher H, et al. COL4A4 mutation in thin basement membrane disease previously described in Alport syndrome. Kidney Int 60:480–483, 2001.
24. Nieuwhof CMG, de Heer F, de Leeuw P, van Breda Vriesman PJC. Thin GBM nephropathy: premature glomerular obsolescence is associated with hypertension and late onset renal failure. Kidney Int 51:1596–1601, 1997.

Section IV
Systemic Diseases Affecting the Kidney

8
Lupus Glomerulonephritis

Jan A. Bruijn

Introduction/Clinical Setting

Systemic lupus erythematosus (SLE) is an autoimmune disease of unknown cause that can occur at almost any age, although it affects mostly women in their 20s. The annual incidence of SLE is 50 to 70 people per million of the population, and prevalence is 500 per million (1). Epidemiologic data show that the incidence of new cases and the survival of patients with SLE are both increasing (2). The disease is characterized by a large variety of organ disorders involving many different immune mechanisms. This is reflected in particular by the spectrum of glomerular lesions, resulting in a strong variation of the clinical symptoms of the renal disease. Clinical or morphologic involvement of the kidney in SLE occurs in 50% to 80% of lupus patients at any moment during the course of their disease. Moreover, renal alterations are found in almost 90% of lupus patients at autopsy. The lowest 5-year survival has been reported for patients with central nervous system and renal involvement (1).

The diagnosis of SLE is usually based on the documentation of multisystem involvement that meets at least four of 11 criteria established by the American College of Rheumatology, listed elsewhere (3). The sensitivity and specificity of these criteria are both 96% (3). Clinical signs of lupus nephritis involve most often proteinuria, ranging from minimal to nephrotic and usually correlating with the histologic type of lesion. Membranous and diffuse proliferative forms usually present with proteinuria. Severe glomerular lesions cause hematuria, a telescoped urinary sediment (i.e., red and white blood cells, as well as hyaline, granular, cellular, and broad casts), and renal insufficiency that may rapidly lead to complete loss of renal function. Hypertension usually develops later in the course of the disease.

Classification of the renal pathology of lupus patients is based on light microscopic changes, combined with immunohistochemical and ultrastructural observations. The classification was most recently revised in 2003 by a working group under the auspices of the Renal Pathology

TABLE 8.1. 2003 International Society of Nephrology/Renal Pathology Society (ISN/RPS) classification of lupus glomerulonephritis (LGN) (4)

Class I: minimal mesangial lupus nephritis

Normal glomeruli by light microscopy (LM), but mesangial immune deposits by immunofluorescence (IF) and/or electron microscopy (EM)

Class II: mesangial proliferative lupus nephritis

Purely mesangial hypercellularity of any degree or mesangial matrix expansion by LM with mesangial immune deposits; may be a few isolated subepithelial and/or subendothelial deposits by IF and/or EM, but not visible by LM

Class III: focal lupus nephritis[a]

Active or inactive focal, segmental or global endo- or extracapillary glomerulonephritis involving <50% of all glomeruli, typically with focal subendothelial immune deposits, with or without mesangial alterations

III (A) Active lesions: *focal proliferative LGN*
III (A/C) Active and chronic lesions: *focal proliferative and sclerosing LGN*
III (C) Chronic inactive lesions with glomerular scars: *focal sclerosing LGN*

Class IV: diffuse lupus nephritis[b]

Active or inactive diffuse, segmental or global endo- or extracapillary glomerulonephritis involving ≥50% of all glomeruli, typically with diffuse subendothelial immune deposits, with or without mesangial alterations. This class is divided into diffuse segmental (IV-S) lupus nephritis when ≥50% of the involved glomeruli have segmental lesions, and diffuse global (IV-G) lupus nephritis when ≥50% of the involved glomeruli have global lesions.

Segmental is defined as a glomerular lesion that involves less than half of the glomerular tuft. This class includes cases with diffus wire loop deposits but with little or no glomerular proliferation.

IV-S (A) Active lesions: *diffuse segmental proliferative lupus nephritis*
IV-G (A) Active lesions: *diffuse global proliferative lupus nephritis*
IV-S (A/C) Active and chronic lesions: *diffuse segmental proliferative and sclerosing lupus nephritis*
IV-G (A/C) Active and chronic lesions: *diffuse global proliferative and sclerosing lupus nephritis*
IV-S (C) Chronic inactive lesions with scars: *diffuse segmental sclerosing lupus nephritis*
IV-G (C) Chronic inactive lesions with scars: *diffuse global sclerosing lupus nephritis*

Class V: membranous lupus nephritis

Global or segmental subepithelial immune deposits or their morphologic sequelae by LM and by IF or EM, with or without mesangial alterations

Class V lupus nephritis may occur in combination with class III or IV, in which case both will be diagnosed

Class V may show advanced sclerosis

Class VI: advanced sclerosing lupus nephritis

>90% of glomeruli globally sclerosed without residual activity

[a] Indicate the proportion of glomeruli with active and with sclerotic lesions.
[b] Indicate the proportion of glomeruli with fibrinoid necrosis and/or cellular crescents.
Note: Indicate the grade (mild, moderate, severe), tubular atrophy, interstitial inflammation and fibrosis, severity of arteriosclerosis, or other vascular lesions.

TABLE 8.2. Abbreviated ISN/RPS classification of lupus nephritis (2003)

Class I	Minimal mesangial lupus nephritis
Class II	Mesangial proliferative lupus nephritis
Class III	Focal lupus nephritis[a]
Class IV	Diffuse segmental (IV-S) or global (IV-G) lupus nephritis[b]
Class V	Membranous lupus nephritis[c]
Class VI	Advanced sclerosing lupus nephritis

[a] Indicate the proportion of glomeruli with active and with sclerotic lesions.
[b] Indicate the proportion of glomeruli with fibrinoid necrosis and/or cellular crescents.
[c] Class V may occur in combination with class III or IV, in which case both will be diagnosed.
Note: Indicate the grade (mild, moderate, severe), tubular atrophy, interstitial inflammation and fibrosis, severity of arteriosclerosis, or other vascular lesions.

TABLE 8.3. Definition of active and chronic glomerular lesions according to the 2003 ISN/RPS classification of lupus nephritis

Active lesions
Endocapillary hypercellularity with or without leukocyte infiltration and with substantial luminal reduction
Karyorrhexis
Fibrinoid necrosis
Rupture of glomerular basement membrane
Crescents, cellular or fibrocellular
Subendothelial deposits identifiable by LM (wire loops)
Intraluminal immune aggregates (hyaline thrombi)
Chronic lesions
Glomerular sclerosis (segmental, global)
Fibrous adhesions
Fibrous crescents

Society (RPS) and the International Society of Nephrology (ISN) (Tables 8.1 to 8.3) (4).

Pathologic Findings

Light Microscopy, Immunofluorescence, and Electron Microscopy

Lupus Nephritis Classes I and II

Classes I and II lupus nephritis refer to pure mesangial glomerulopathy. These patients present clinically with mild hematuria, or proteinuria, or

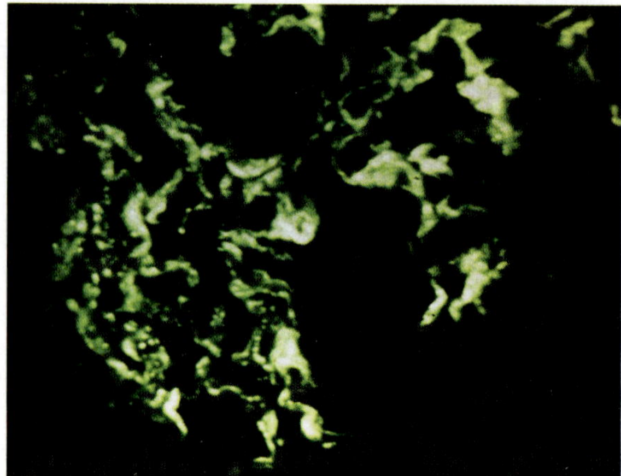

FIGURE 8.1. Lupus nephritis ISN/RPS class II (mesangial) with granular mesangial immunoglobulin G (IgG) (immunofluorescence).

both. In general they have a good prognosis with respect to their renal function, and the histologic alterations remain stable in the majority of cases. However, functional deterioration and progression of glomerular lesions to more active or generalized proliferative forms occurs in about 20% of cases. In the past decades the availability of better supportive therapy and more selective use of immunosuppressive agents has led to improved survival of patients with mild forms of lupus glomerulonephritis, while new forms of immunosuppressive therapy are being developed (5,6).

Class I or minimal mesangial lupus glomerulonephritis refers to biopsies showing normal glomeruli by light microscopy, but mesangial immune deposits by immunofluorescence or electron microscopy. Class II contains mesangial proliferative lesions characterized by purely mesangial hypercellularity of any degree or mesangial matrix expansion by light microscopy with immune deposits, predominantly mesangial with none or few isolated subepithelial or subendothelial deposits by immunfluorescence or electron microscopy but not visible by light microscopy (Fig. 8.1).

Lupus Nephritis Class III

Class III lupus nephritis entails *focal* (involving less than half of the glomeruli available for inspection) and *segmental* (involving mostly a small part or a segment of the cut surface of the affected glomeruli) or *global* (involving the majority of the cut surface of the involved glomeruli) proliferative, necrotizing, or sclerosing lesions. The involvement of the glomeruli may occur in different combinations. A subdivision is made according to the predominance of active versus sclerotic lesions as indicated in Table 8.1.

In the pathology report, the proportion of glomeruli with active and with sclerotic lesions and the proportion of glomeruli with fibrinoid necrosis or cellular crescents should be indicated. The lesions may be superimposed on a diffuse mesangial expansion, as seen in class II lupus nephritis. Narrowing and obliteration of the capillary lumina is often present with segmental intracapillary and extracapillary proliferation and adhesions of visceral and parietal epithelial cells (Figs. 8.2 and 8.3). In addition, nuclear debris is seen as well as influx of inflammatory cells, which has been ascribed to altered expression of adhesion molecules in the diseased vessel walls (7,8). The inflammatory process may also lead to disruption of the glomerular basement membrane and fibrinoid necrosis. Amorphous eosinophilic material staining bright red in trichrome staining and present most often in the context of an extracapillary proliferative lesion is regarded as fibrinoid necrosis. However, little is known about the pathogenesis, specificity, and molecular content of fibrinoid necrosis, although splice variants of fibronectin seem to be present in the lesion (9–11). In the affected glomerular areas, endothelial damage may allow direct contact between serum proteins and collagen present in the subendothelial basement membrane, leading to activation of the coagulation cascade. Thus, necrotizing lesions may contain fibrin or microthrombi. Segmental sclerotic scars with capsule adhesions can develop from focal crescents with necrotic lesions. Focal tubular and interstitial signs of nephron deterioration can be seen. The validity of the cutoff point between classes III and IV of 50% involved glomeruli has been disputed recently, but is currently retained in the 2003 revision of the lupus nephritis classification system (4,12).

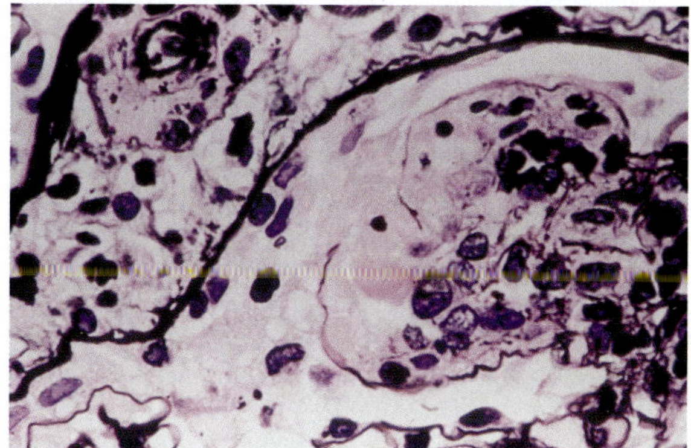

Figure 8.2. Lupus nephritis ISN/RPS class III, focal proliferative: early necrotizing lesion with rupture of glomerular basement membrane (Jones silver stain).

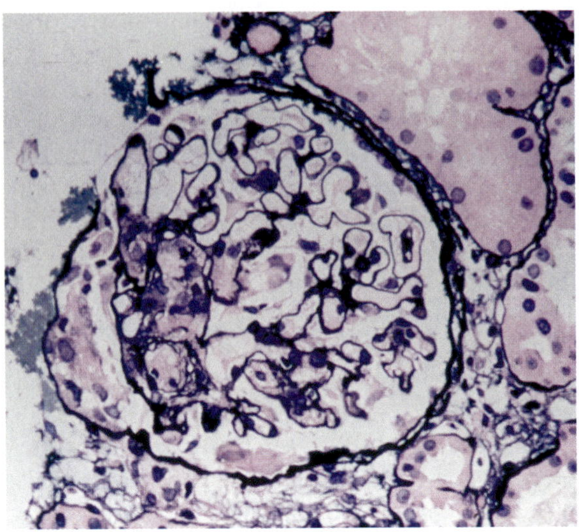

FIGURE 8.3. Lupus nephritis ISN/RPS class III, focal proliferative: segmental proliferative lesion ("crescent") (Jones silver stain).

Immunofluorescence investigations show the presence of immunoglobulin G (IgG), IgM, and IgA immunoglobulins, complement factors C3 and C1q ("full-house" immunofluorescence) in granular and globular depositions along the glomerular capillary walls and in the mesangium (Fig. 8.4). Although the light microscopic changes are focal, the immunofluorescence

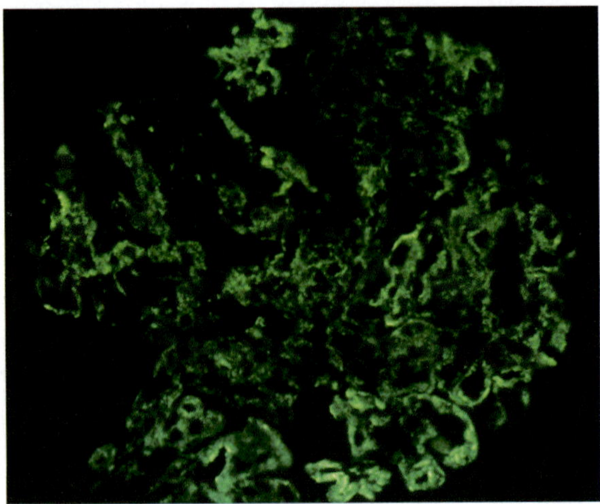

FIGURE 8.4. Lupus nephritis ISN/RPS class III, focal proliferative: diffuse, chunky granular pattern for IgG (immunofluorescence).

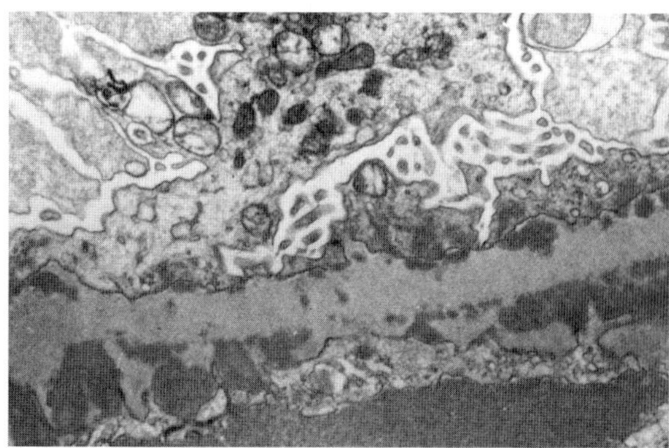

FIGURE 8.5. Subendothelial and subepithelial electron-dense deposits along the glomerular basement membrane (GBM) with irregular thickenings of GBM and pseudovillous transformation of visceral epithelial cells in lupus nephritis ISN/RPS class III lupus nephritis (electron microscopy).

is in most cases positive in all glomeruli. Electron microscopy typically demonstrates deposits in the mesangium and in about half of the cases also subendothelially or subepithelially along the glomerular basement membranes (Fig. 8.5) (13).

Patients with lupus nephritis class III present almost invariably with proteinuria, and in the majority of cases with nephrotic syndrome. The lesions can progress to diffuse proliferative (class IV) or membranous lupus glomerulonephritis. Progression is possibly predicted by the presence of subendothelial and subepithelial deposits.

Lupus Nephritis Class IV

Class IV, the most common and severe form of lupus nephritis, refers to *diffuse segmental* (IV-S) or *global* (IV-G) proliferative forms of glomerulonephritis, characterized by diffuse hypercellularity in more than 50% of the glomeruli. The lesions may be either active or inactive, have a segmental or global distribution, and may manifest endo- or extracapillary glomerulonephritis with diffuse subendothelial immune deposits, with or without mesangial alterations. Some investigators revealed the poor outcome of diffuse segmental necrotizing glomerulonephritis involving over 50% of glomeruli (which these investigators consider a severe form of class III), as compared to other forms of class IV lupus nephritis (14). Class IV, therefore, is divided into diffuse segmental (IV-S) when ≥50% of the involved glomeruli have segmental lesions, and diffuse global (IV-G) when ≥50% of the involved glomeruli have global lesions (Fig. 8.6) (4). Furthermore, a subdivision is made according to the presence of active versus chronic lesions as was indicated for class III lesions (Table 8.1).

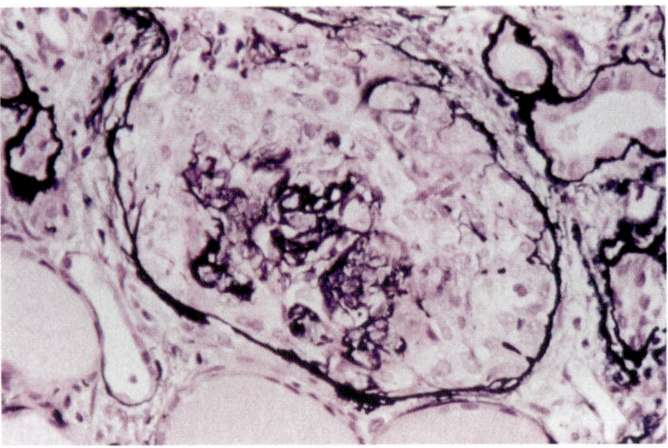

FIGURE 8.6. Circumferential ("global") extracapillary proliferation ("crescent") in ISN/RPS class IV diffuse proliferative lupus nephritis (Jones silver stain).

As in class III, in the pathology report the proportion of glomeruli with active and with sclerotic lesions and the proportion of glomeruli with fibrinoid necrosis or cellular crescents should be indicated. Between the proliferating cells focal fibrinoid necrosis is often seen with capillary mural thrombi or perforation of the glomerular capillary walls. In addition, *hematoxylin bodies* may be seen, representing nuclei altered by antinuclear antibodies. "*Wire-loop*" *lesions*, that is, local periodic acid-Schiff (PAS)-positive thickenings of the glomerular capillary walls, are characteristic of this form of lupus nephritis (Fig. 8.7). This thickening of the capillary walls is related to the presence of large, mostly subendothelial electron dense deposits. Glomerular lesions run the gamut from diffuse hypercellularity

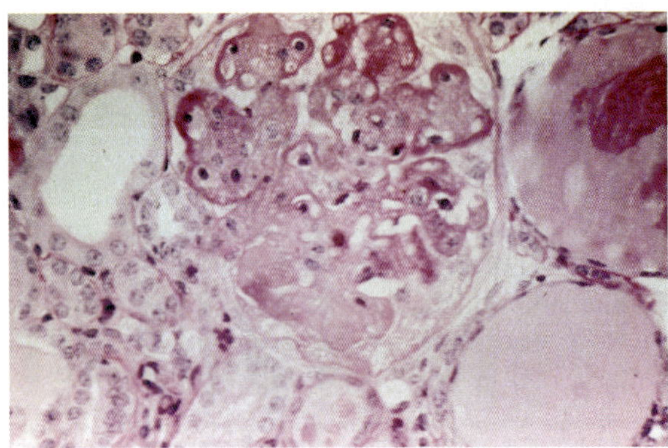

FIGURE 8.7. Glomerulus in ISN/RPS class IV diffuse proliferative lupus nephritis: sclerosing lesion and "wire loops" [periodic acid-Schiff (PAS) stain].

to severe necrotizing "crescentic" glomerulonephritis or, in chronic cases, diffuse global glomerulosclerosis with loss of renal function. Formation of "spikes" along the glomerular basement membrane can be seen, as well as lobular accentuation of the glomerular architecture and "interpositioning" of mesangial cells along the glomerular capillary walls, giving rise to the picture of membranoproliferative glomerulonephritis. In these cases proliferating mesangial cells extend along the inner side of the glomerular capillary wall, depositing new extracellular matrix on the lumenal side, leading to double contours of the basement membrane. Whether lobular or membranoproliferative lupus glomerulonephritis should be regarded as a separate entity is unclear, but intermediate forms of lobular and diffuse proliferative glomerular lesions may occur. Tubular and interstitial signs of nephron deterioration are more extensive in class IV than in class III lupus nephritis. The predictive value of these lesions with respect to renal function, however, is disputed (15,16). The tubular epithelium shows cytoplasmic hyaline droplets, hydropic degeneration, cytoplasmic vacuolization, hyalin protein cylinders, and, in more advanced, glomerulosclerotic stages of the disease tubular atrophy and interstitial fibrosis. Arteries and arterioles usually show no pathologic changes.

Immunofluorescence in lupus nephritis class IV shows irregular deposits of immunoglobulins and complement along the glomerular capillary walls and in the mesangium (Fig. 8.8). Ultrastructurally, electron dense deposits are seen in the mesangium and subendothelially along the capillary walls, in larger quantities than in the other classes. Proliferating mesangial cells extending along the inner side of peripheral capillary walls and incorporation of subendothelial deposits can be seen by electron microscopy as well. Deposits are usually also present intramembranously and subepithelially, with obliteration of epithelial foot processes. In addition, epithelial cells

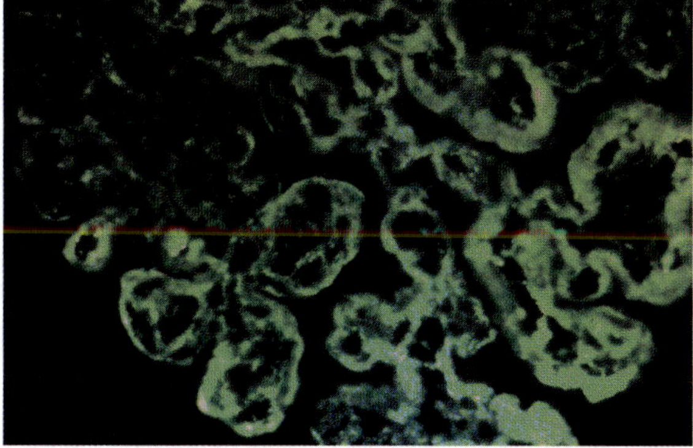

FIGURE 8.8. Lupus nephritis ISN/RPS class IV diffuse proliferative: large confluent predominantly subendothelial IgG deposits along GBM (immunofluorescence).

may be enlarged and show pseudovillous transformation with increase of cytoplasmic organelles. Microtubular *myxovirus-like particles* or *tubuloreticular inclusions* (TRIs) can be found in the cytoplasm of endothelial cells or lymphocytes, localized in dilated segments of rough and smooth endoplasmic reticulum. These TRIs are not specific for SLE but are often seen in patients with AIDS and other viral infections, probably reflecting local or systemic α-interferon production. Large and often confluent subendothelial deposits represent the ultrastructural analogue of the "wire-loop" lesions seen light microscopically. Subepithelial deposits can be large, as in acute proliferative glomerulonephritis. Penetration of the subepithelial deposits in the underlying basement membrane and partial embracement of the deposits by the spike-like basement membrane thickenings are often present. As in the other classes of lupus nephritis, the electron dense deposits can show a typical fingerprint-like crystalline pattern, considered pathognomonic for lupus nephritis and possibly representing the presence of cryoglobulins.

Patients with class IV lupus nephritis may show a rapidly progressive renal failure with high proteinuria and, without treatment, a poor prognosis with respect to renal function.

Lupus Nephritis Class V

Class V lupus nephritis is characterized by diffuse membranous glomerulonephritis. Among patients with lupus nephritis the incidence of membranous glomerulonephritis varies between 8% and 27%. The prognosis of patients with membranous lupus nephritis is relatively favorable, with a reported 10-year kidney survival of 91% (17). Still, one third of patients with membranous lupus nephritis progress to proliferative lupus nephritis (18). Characteristically patients present with high proteinuria at an early stage. By light microscopy, some mesangial expansion is seen with diffuse thickening of the glomerular capillary walls in hematoxylin and eosin (H&E) and PAS stains. With silver-methenamine staining, argyrophilic spike-like formations often can be seen in subepithelial locations along the glomerular basement membrane. The spikes correspond to thickenings of the basement membrane between and around the subepithelially localized immune deposits, as can be seen by electron microscopy. Altered basement membrane homeostasis probably underlies the spike formation (13). By immunofluorescence, granular deposits of immunoglobulins and complement are usually present in the mesangium and peripherally along the glomerular capillary walls, corresponding to the presence of subepithelial electron dense deposits. In addition to IgG and C3, the presence of IgA and C1q in the deposits is regarded as a marker for lupus membranous glomerulonephritis (19), although the presence of IgA and C1q has also been noted in idiopathic membranous glomerulopathy. The deposits in membranous lupus nephritis are usually regularly distributed and uniform in size. This in contrast to proliferative lupus nephritis, in which the deposits are irregularly distributed and of differing size. Epithelial cells show extensive obliteration of foot processes. Although similar stages of development can be seen in class V lupus nephritis as in idiopathic membranous glomerulopathy, in lupus nephritis mesangial deposits are more often present.

Class V lupus nephritis may occur in combination with classes III or IV in which case both are diagnosed. The presence of subendothelial deposits or necrosis is probably of more prognostic value than a coinciding membranous pattern: patients with pure membranous lupus nephritis experience a relatively benign course, whereas in those with mixed membranous and diffuse proliferative lesions, the survival rates are similar to those of patients with diffuse lupus nephritis alone. Likewise, in a study of membranous lupus nephritis, patients with a major endocapillary proliferative component had higher serum creatinine levels at entry and were more likely to experience a decline in renal function than those without proliferation (20).

Lupus Nephritis Class VI

This class refers to a late stage, resembling morphologically any late or end stage in chronic glomerulonephritis with global sclerosis of >90% of glomeruli without residual activity. Alternatively or in addition, secondary focal and segmental glomerulosclerosis with its different subtypes may develop (21). Specific features for lupus nephritis are usually lacking. However, in patients with lupus nephritis such chronic end-stage glomerulosclerotic lesions are seldom seen. Patients with lupus nephritis who have been treated for longer periods may show chronic glomerular lesions at autopsy. These may be morphologically similar to other late stages of glomerulonephritis and of focal global sclerotic lesions that occur invariably at an older age (22).

Etiology/Pathogenesis

Investigations of human biopsies together with research using animal models and in vitro cell culture systems have generated some understanding of the underlying etiologic and pathogenetic mechanisms of lupus nephritis (23–27). The findings indicate that disturbed Fas-FasL–mediated apoptosis is a cause of autoimmunity in SLE (28–31). Subsequent breakdown in immunologic tolerance leads to the production of autoreactive B and T cells that, through either direct infiltration or their secretory products, initiate inflammation (32). Selective polyclonal B-cell expansion possibly related to disturbances in the idiotype network and genetic factors may be of primary importance in the initiation and development of autoimmunity as well (25,33–36). For example, the Fc gamma RIIIA-V/F158 gene polymorphism has a significant impact on the development of lupus nephritis (37). Intriguingly, SLE and lupus nephritis have also been described in patients with autoimmune phenomena after infection with the human immunodeficiency virus (HIV) (38). Among the molecules identified as target antigens of pathogenetic autoantibodies in lupus nephritis are single-stranded and double-stranded DNA, nucleosomes, C1q, visceral epithelial cell surface antigens, and basement membrane components such as laminin (25,39–44). Antiphospholipid antibodies have been detected in 25% to 50% of SLE patients, some of whom develop lupus anticoagulant or antiphospholipid syndrome with clinical signs of thrombosis (45–47).

Within the spectrum of lupus nephritis different tissue reactions occur, each leading to a different type of renal lesion both clinically and morphologically. Although lymphokines, cytokines, and other cellular factors contribute to the inflammation and subsequent fibrosis, the site where the immune complexes deposit is of primary concern in the pathogenesis of the disease because different glomerular localizations of complexes initiate different pathogenetic pathways (48). The localization of the complexes is determined by the specificity, affinity, and avidity of the antibodies formed, their class and subclass, and the size and valence of the complexes (23,49,50). In general, when an immune reaction is characterized by the presence of relatively small amounts of stable, intermediate-sized complexes formed with high-affinity antibodies, it is likely to result in mesangial glomerulonephritis. These complexes accumulate in the mesangium as part of filtration residues, which may be cleared adequately by the mesangial clearing system, resulting in mild glomerular lesions. With larger complexes formed by high-avidity antibodies, or with larger numbers of complexes, the capacity of the mesangium to handle macromolecules becomes overloaded, resulting in a subendothelial accumulation of these complexes as well. The subendothelial complexes are able to activate circulating inflammatory mediators, especially the complement system (7). Adhesion molecules are then upregulated and inflammatory cells arrested and activated (51). The interaction between particular antibodies and endothelial cell surface integrins via fibronectin may be involved in their subsequent internalization by endothelial cells (52). This leads to a more severe, diffuse histopathologic lesion with cell proliferation and, possibly, necrosis. Alternatively, an immune response may lead to the occurrence of small, unstable immune complexes formed by low-avidity or low-affinity antibodies in the presence of antigen excess. These complexes may dissociate, followed by reassociation subepithelially and the development of a membranous type of glomerulopathy. Subepithelial complexes can activate complement, but chemotaxis is frustrated by the inability of inflammatory cells to pass the glomerular basement membrane. Thus a prolonged, chronic inflammation occurs, eventually leading to abnormal basement membrane production, increased basement membrane permeability, proteinuria, and a nephrotic syndrome. Proteinuria causes further damage to podocytes with loss of slit-diaphragm proteins and effacement of foot processes (53).

The pathogenesis of glomerulosclerosis in lupus nephritis has in recent years been the subject of a number of investigations, which showed that abnormal homeostasis of matrix and growth factors due to immunologic and hemodynamic factors is probably the underlying cause (22,54–58). In experimental models, aberrant homeostasis of glomerular matrix is associated with glomerular influx of inflammatory cells (59). It is characterized by the occurrence of intramolecular changes of matrix molecules due to alternative splicing of mRNA, chain-specific alterations in synthesis, and neoexpression of matrix epitopes and of adhesion sites that mediate the accumulation of matrix and the influx of inflammatory cells (56,60–63). Interference with such adhesion processes has been effective therapeutically in animal models (59,64). Current investigations are directed at the use of gene polymorphisms and RNA changes as predictors of glomerulosclerosis, allowing early therapeutic and preventive intervention (65–70). This strategy has already proven successful in experimental circumstances (71).

Because of their clinical consequences, the classification of lupus nephritis is based on these distinctive pathogenetic pathways with their accompanying morphologic patterns.

Clinicopathologic Correlations

Classification of lupus nephritis is considered useful to describe the patient's clinical status and for grouping patients with similar clinical profiles. Moreover, the classification is related to prognosis with respect to renal function and patient survival (40). It has been generally accepted that the use of the lupus nephritis classification facilitates the ease and reliability with which nephrologists and nephropathologists communicate information, and that it has greatly improved standardization and reproducibility of biopsy interpretation (45). In contrast, the prognostic value of the so-called activity and chronicity indices used by some in lupus nephritis is subject to discussion, and the utility of these indices is limited by concerns about their irreproducibility (15–17,72). Nevertheless, distinguishing "active" and "sclerosing" lesions (Table 8.3) may help determine prognosis and sensitivity to treatment in both lupus and other glomerulonephritides (73–76). In general, lesions that are potentially sensitive to treatment and reversible show activity, characterized by hypercellularity, leukocyte exudation, necrosis/karyorrhexis, cellular crescents, hyalin deposits, and interstitial inflammatory infiltrate. Renal thrombotic microangiopathy during SLE may be treatable with plasmapheresis similar to primary hemolytic uremic syndrome or thrombotic thrombocytopenic purpura (77). More permanent lesions less sensitive to treatment are glomerulosclerosis, fibrous crescents, tubular atrophy, and interstitial fibrosis (78). At the ultrastructural level the presence of subendothelial deposits is generally regarded as unfavorable. The persistence of subendothelial deposits has been associated with the progression of lupus nephritis and the decrease in the amount of subendothelial and mesangial deposits with a lower risk for renal impairment in SLE. Therefore, the existing inverse relationship of glomerular deposits and macrophage influx would help account for the previous demonstration of the association of glomerular macrophage infiltration with improved renal prognosis (79).

Studying the kidney biopsy thus helps to distinguish potentially treatable from untreatable renal disorders and to determine the patient's prognosis with respect to renal function, especially within the group of proliferative lupus nephritides (80–83). Although lupus nephritis encompasses a number of different glomerular lesions, the type of glomerular lesion remains unchanged in about half of the cases. In the other half transformation occurs to either more ominous or more benign histologic patterns, the latter particularly under the influence of therapy. Patients have been described with apparently severe kidney disease, in which renal function and morphologic alterations remained stable for a longer period, whereas other patients with apparently mild forms of lupus nephritis showed rapid progression to severe renal disease with loss of renal function. In patients with the most severe forms of lupus nephritis, a remission of clinical renal abnormalities is associated with dramatic improvement in long-term patient and renal survival (84). With current management strategies, in general the long-term outlook for patients with lupus nephritis has improved, but only a minority of patients are able to stop treatment altogether, and the incidence of serious complications is high (78,85–93); infection being the leading cause of death (94). Long-term courses of intravenous cyclophosphamide with a cumulative risk of toxicity are advocated to achieve remission in many first-treated patients and in most patients treated for a second time (95–97). Alternatively, for patients with proliferative lupus nephritis, short-term therapy with intravenous cyclophosphamide followed by maintenance therapy with mycophenolate mofetil or azathioprine appears to be more efficacious and safer than long-term therapy with intravenous cyclophosphamide (98,99). Overall only 10% to 15% of patients with lupus nephritis now go into end-stage renal failure (40). In these patients clinical and serologic SLE activity may persist (100).

References

1. Picken MM. The role of kidney biopsy in the management of patients with systemic lupus erythematosus. Pathol Case Rev 3:204–209, 1998.
2. Ruiz-Irastorza G, Khamashta MA, Castellino G, Hughes GRV. Systemic lupus erythematosus. Lancet 357:1027–1032, 2001.

3. Bloom BJ, Bramson RT, Weinstein HJ, Pasternack MS, Zukerberg LR. Weekly clinicopathological exercise: systemic lupus erythematosus. N Engl J Med 340:1491–1497, 1999.
4. Weening JJ, d'Agati VD, Schwartz MM, et al. The classification of glomerulonephritis in systemic lupus erythematosus revisited. J Am Soc Nephrol 15:241–250, 2004.
5. Donadio JV, Jr, Glassock RJ. Immunosuppressive drug therapy in lupus nephritis. Am J Kidney Dis 21:239–250, 1993.
6. Entani C, Izumino K, Iida H, et al. Effect of a novel immunosuppressant, FK506, on spontaneous lupus nephritis in MRL/MpJ-lpr/lpr mice. Nephron 64:471–475, 1993.
7. Marinides GN, Border WA. Nephritogenic immune reactions involving planted renal antigens. In: Massry SG, Glassock RJ, eds. Textbook of Nephrology, 3rd ed. Baltimore: Williams & Wilkins, 1995:631–635.
8. Bruijn JA, Dinklo NJCM. Distinct patterns of expression of intercellular adhesion molecule-1, vascular cell adhesion molecule-1, and endothelial-leukocyte adhesion molecule-1, in renal disease. Lab Invest 69:329–335, 1993.
9. Bajema IM, Bruijn JA. What stuff is this! A historical perspective on fibrinoid necrosis. J Pathol 191:235–238, 2000.
10. Bajema IM, Hagen EC, de Heer E, van der Woude FJ, Bruijn JA. Colocalization of ANCA-antigens and fibrinoid necrosis in ANCA-associated vasculitis. Kidney Int 60:2025–2030, 2001.
11. Bajema IM, Hagen EC, Ferrario F, de Heer E, Bruijn JA. Immunopathological aspects of systemic vasculitis. Springer Semin Immunopathol 23:253–265, 2001.
12. Bruijn JA, Verburgh CA, Huizinga TW. Classifying lupus nephritis. A 32-year-old woman with systemic lupus erythematosus and nephritic syndrome. Am J Kidney Dis 37:653–657, 2001.
13. Bruijn JA. The glomerular basement membrane in lupus nephritis. Microsc Res Techn 28:178–192, 1994.
14. Najafi CC, Korbet SM, Lewis EJ, Schwartz MM, Reichlin M, Evans J. Significance of histologic patterns of glomerular injury upon long-term prognosis in severe lupus glomerulonephritis. Kidney Int 59:2156–2163, 2001.
15. Schwartz MM, Lan S-P, Bernstein J, Hill GS, Holley K, Lewis EJ, Lupus Nephritis Collaboration Study Group. Role of pathology indices in the management of severe lupus glomerulonephritis. Kidney Int 42:743–748, 1992.
16. Schwartz MM, Lan S, Bernstein J, Hill GS, Holley K, Lewis EJ, Lupus Nephritis Collaboration Study Group. Irreproducibility of the activity and chronicity indices limits their utility in the management of lupus nephritis. Am J Kidney Dis 21:374–377, 1993.
17. Pasquali S, Banfi G, Zucchelli A, Moroni G, Ponticelli C, Zucchelli P. Lupus membranous nephropathy: long-term outcome. Clin Nephrol 39:175–182, 1993.
18. Mercadel L, Tezenas du Montcel S, Nochy D, et al. Factors affecting outcome and prognosis in membranous lupus nephropathy. Nephrol Dial Transplant 17:1771–1778, 2002.
19. Haas M, Zikos D. Membranous nephropathy. Distinction of latent membranous lupus nephritis from idiopathic membranous nephropathy on renal biopsy. Pathol Case Rev 3:175–179, 1998.

20. Schwartz MM, Kawala K, Roberts JL, Humes C, Lewis EJ. Clinical and pathological features of membranous glomerulonephritis of systemic lupus erythematosus. Am J Nephrol 4:301–311, 1984.
21. D'Agati V, Fogo AB, Bruijn JA, Jennette JC. Pathologic classification of focal segmental glomerulosclerosis: a working proposal. Am J Kidney Dis 2:368–382, 2004.
22. Bruijn JA, Cotran RS. The aging kidney: pathologic alterations. In: Martinez-Maldonado M, ed. Hypertension and Renal Disease in the Elderly. Boston: Blackwell Scientific, 1992:1–10.
23. Bruijn JA, Hoedemaeker PJ. Nephritogenic immune reactions involving native renal antigens. In: Massry SG, Glassock RJ, eds. Textbook of Nephrology, 3rd ed. Baltimore: Williams & Wilkins, 1995:627–631.
24. Bruijn JA, Bergijk EC, de Heer E, Fleuren GJ, Hoedemaeker PJ. Induction and progression of experimental lupus nephritis: exploration of a pathogenetic pathway. Kidney Int 41:5–13, 1992.
25. Hahn BH. Antibodies to DNA. N Engl J Med 338:1359–1368, 1998.
26. Herrmann M, Voll RE, Kalden JR. Etiopathogenesis of systemic lupus erythematosus. Immunol Today 21:424–426, 2000.
27. Peutz-Kootstra CJ, de Heer E, Hoedemaeker PhJ, Abrass CK, Bruijn JA. Lupus nephritis: lessons from experimental animals. J Lab Clin Med 137:244–260, 2001.
28. Tax WJM, Kramers C, van Bruggen MCJ, Berden JHM. Apoptosis, nucleosomes, and nephritis in systemic lupus erythematosus. Kidney Int 48: 666–673, 1995.
29. Berden JHM. Lupus nephritis. Kidney Int 52:538–558, 1997.
30. Wada T, Schwarting A, Kinoshita K, et al. Fas on renal parenchymal cells does not promote autoimmune nephritis in MRL mice. Kidney Int 55:841–851, 1999.
31. Salmon M, Gordon C. The role of apoptosis in systemic lupus erythematosus. Rheumatology 38:1177–1183, 1999.
32. Su W, Madaio MP. Recent advances in the pathogenesis of lupus nephritis: autoantibodies and B cells. Semin Nephrol 23:564–568, 2003.
33. Sutmuller M, Baelde JJ, Madaio MP, Bruijn JA, de Heer E. Idiotype usage by polyclonally activated B cells in experimental autoimmunity and infection. Clin Exp Immunol 115:275–280, 1999.
34. Sutmuller M, Baelde HJ, Ouellette S, de Heer E, Bruijn JA. T-cell receptor Vβ gene expression in experimental lupus nephritis. Immunology 95:18–25, 1998.
35. Hopkinson ND, Jenkinson C, Muir KR, Doherty M, Powell RJ. Racial group, socioeconomic status, and the development of persistent proteinuria in systemic lupus erythematosus. Ann Rheum Dis 59:116–119, 2000.
36. Kaliyaperumal A, Michaels MA, Datta SK. Naturally processed chromatin peptides reveal a major autoepitope that primes pathogenic T and B cells of lupus. J Immunol 168:2530–2537, 2002.
37. Karassa FB, Trikalinos TA, Ioannidis JP. The Fc gamma RIIIA-F158 allele is a risk factor for the development of lupus nephritis: a meta-analysis. Kidney Int 63:1475–1482, 2003.

38. Chang BG, Markowitz GS, Seshan SV, Seigle RL, D'Agati VD. Renal manifestations of concurrent systemic lupus erythematosus and HIV infection. Am J Kidney Dis 33:441–449, 1999.
39. Coremans IEM, Bruijn JA, de Heer E, Van der Voort EAM, Breedveld FC, Daha MR. Stabilization of glomerular deposits of C1q by antibodies against C1q in mice. J Clin Lab Immunol 44:47–61, 1995.
40. Cameron JS. Lupus nephritis. J Am Soc Nephrol 10:413–424, 1999.
41. Kootstra CJ, Veninga A, Baelde JJ, van Eendenburg J, de Heer E, Bruijn JA. Characterization of reactivity of monoclonal autoantibodies with renal antigens in experimental lupus nephritis. J Clin Lab Immunol 48:201–218, 1996.
42. Van Leer EHG, Bruijn JA, Prins FA, Hoedemaeker PJ, de Heer E. Redistribution of glomerular dipeptidyl peptidase type IV in experimental lupus nephritis. Lab Invest 68:550–556, 1993.
43. Mostoslavsky G, Fischel R, Yachimovich N, et al. Lupus anti-DNA autoantibodies cross-react with a glomerular structural protein: a case for tissue injury by molecular mimicry. Eur J Immunol 21:1221–1227, 2001.
44. Licht R, van Bruggen MC, Oppers-Walgreen B, Rijke TB, Berden JH. Plasma levels of nucleosomes and nucleosome-autoantibody complexes in murine lupus: effects of disease progression and lipopolysaccharide administration. Arthritis Rheum 44:1320–1330, 2001.
45. D'Agati V. Renal disease in systemic lupus erythematosus, mixed connective tissue disease, Sjögren's syndrome, and rheumatoid arthritis. In: Jennette JC, Olson JL, Schwartz MM, Silva FG, eds. Heptinstall's Pathology of the Kidney, 5th ed. Philadelphia: Lippincott-Raven, 1998:541–624.
46. Rennke HG, Fang LS-T, Laposata M. Antiphospholipid-antibody syndrome. N Engl J Med 340:900–1908, 1999.
47. Fialova L, Zima T, Tesar V, et al. Antiphospholipid antibodies in patients with lupus nephritis. Ren Fail 25:747–758, 2003.
48. Madaio MP, McLoud TC, McCluskey RT. Weekly clinicopathological exercise: lupus nephritis. N Engl J Med 338:1308–1317, 1998.
49. Bruijn JA, de Heer E, Hoedemaeker PJ. Immune mechanisms in injury to glomeruli and tubulo-interstitial tissue. In: Jones TC, ed. Monographs on Pathology of Laboratory Animals. Urinary System, 2nd ed. New York: Springer-Verlag, 1998:199–224.
50. Hogendoorn PCW, van Dorst EBL, van der Burg SH, et al. Antigen size influences the type of glomerular pathology in chronic serum sickness. Nephrol Dial Transplant 8:703–710, 1993.
51. Bruijn JA, de Heer E. Biology of disease. Adhesion molecules in renal diseases. Lab Invest 72:387–394, 1995.
52. Fujii H, Nakatani K, Arita N, et al. Internalization of antibodies by endothelial cells via fibronectin implicating a novel mechanism in lupus nephritis. Kidney Int 64:1662–1670, 2003.
53. Koop K, Eikmans M, Baelde HJ, et al. Expression of podocyte-associated molecules in acquired human kidney diseases. J Am Soc Nephrol 14:2063–2071, 2003.
54. Hricik DE, Chung-Park M, Sedor JR. Glomerulonephritis. N Engl J Med 339:888–900, 1998.

55. Bruijn JA, Roos A, de Geus B, de Heer E. Transforming growth factor-b and the glomerular extracellular matrix in renal pathology. J Lab Clin Med 123:34–47, 1994.
56. Bergijk EC, de Heer E, Hoedemaeker PJ, Bruijn JA. A reappraisal of immune-mediated glomerulosclerosis. A review. Kidney Int 49:605–611, 1996.
57. Remuzzi G, Bertani T. Pathophysiology of progressive nephropathies. N Engl J Med 339:1448–1456, 1998.
58. Van Vliet AI, van Alderwegen IE, Baelde JJ, de Heer E, Bruijn JA. Fibronectin accumulation in glomerulosclerotic lesions. Self-assembly sites and the heparin II binding domain. Kidney Int 61:481–489, 2002.
59. Kootstra CJ, Sutmuller M, Baelde JJ, de Heer E, Bruijn JA. Association between leukocyte infiltration and development of glomerulosclerosis in experimental lupus nephritis. J Pathol 184:219–225, 1998.
60. Bergijk EC, Van Alderwegen IE, Baelde JJ, et al. Differential expression of collagen type IV isoforms in experimental glomerulosclerosis. J Pathol 184:307–315, 1998.
61. Bruijn JA, Kootstra CJ, Sutmuller M, Van Vliet A, Bergijk EC, de Heer E. Matrix and adhesion molecules in kidney pathology: recent observations. J Lab Clin Med 130:357–364, 1997.
62. Bergijk EC, Baelde JJ, Kootstra CJ, de Heer E, Killen PD, Bruijn JA. Cloning of the mouse fibronectin V-region and alteration of its splicing pattern in experimental immunecomplex glomerulonephritis. J Pathol 178:462–468, 1996.
63. Peutz-Kootstra CJ, Hansen K, de Heer E, Abrass CK, Bruijn JA. Differential expression of laminin chains and anti-laminin autoantibodies in experimental lupus nephritis. J Pathol 192:404–412, 2000.
64. Kootstra CJ, van der Giezen DM, Van Krieken JHJM, de Heer E, Bruijn JA. Effective treatment of experimental lupus nephritis by combined administration of anti-CD11a and anti-CD54 antibodies. Clin Exp Immunol 108: 324–332, 1997.
65. Eikmans M, Baelde JJ, de Heer E, Bruijn JA. Processing renal biopsies for diagnostic mRNA quantitation: improvement of RNA extraction and storage conditions. J Am Soc Nephrol 11:868–873, 2000.
66. Eikmans M, Baelde JJ, de Heer E, Bruijn JA. Effect of age and biopsy site on extracellular matrix mRNA and protein levels in human kidney biopsies. Kidney Int 60:974–981, 2001.
67. Rovin BH, Lu L, Zhang X. A novel interleukin-8 polymorphism is associated with severe systemic lupus erythematosus nephritis. Kidney Int 62:261–265, 2002.
68. Eikmans M, Baelde JJ, de Heer E, Bruijn JA. RNA expression profiling as prognostic tool in renal patients: toward nephrogenomics. Kidney Int 62:1125–1135, 2002.
69. Eikmans M, Baelde JJ, de Heer E, Bruijn JA. ECM homeostasis in renal diseases: a genomic approach. J Pathol 200:526–536, 2003.
70. Eikmans M, Baelde HJ, Hagen EC, et al. Renal mRNA levels as prognostic tools in kidney diseases. J Am Soc Nephrol 14:899–907, 2003.
71. Bergijk EC, Baelde HJ, de Heer E, Bruijn JA. Prevention of glomerulosclerosis by early cyclosporine treatment of experimental lupus nephritis. Kidney Int 46:1663–1673, 1994.

72. Austin HA III, Boumpas DT, Vaughan E, Klippel JH, Balow JE. Study of prognostic factors in severe lupus nephritis (LN) [abstract]. J Am Soc Nephrol 3:306, 1992.
73. Bajema IM, Hagen EC, Hermans J, et al. Kidney biopsy as a predictor for renal outcome in ANCA-associated necrotizing glomerulonephritis. Kidney Int 56:1751–1758, 1999.
74. Hauer HA, Bajema IM, van Houwelingen HC, et al. Renal histology in ANCA-associated vasculitis: differences between diagnostic and serologic subgroups. Kidney Int 61:80–89, 2002.
75. Hauer HA, Bajema IM, Hagen EC, et al. Long-term renal injury in ANCA-associated vasculitis: an analysis of 31 patients with follow-up biopsies. Nephrol Dial Transplant 17:587–596, 2002.
76. Yoo CW, Kim M-K, Lee HS. Predictors of renal outcome in diffuse proliferative lupus nephropathy: data from repeat renal biopsy. Nephrol Dial Transplant 15:1604–1608, 2000.
77. Highson MD, Nadasdy T, McCarty GA, Sholer C, Min K-W, Silva F. Renal thrombotic microangiopathy in patients with systemic lupus erythematosus and the antiphospholipid syndrome. Am J Kidney Dis 2:150–158, 1992.
78. Martins L, Rocha G, Rodrigues A, et al. Lupus nephritis: a retrospective review of 78 cases from a single center. Clin Nephrol 57:114–119, 2002.
79. Ichiryu MS, Magil AB. Intraglomerular monocyte infiltration and immune deposits in diffuse lupus glomerulonephritis. Am J Kidney Dis 33:866–871, 1999.
80. Couser WG. Glomerulonephritis. Lancet 353:1509–1515, 1999.
81. Moroni G, Pasquali S, Quaglini S, et al. Clinical and prognostic value of serial renal biopsies in lupus nephritis. Am J Kidney Dis 34:530–539, 1999.
82. Hill GS, Delahousse M, Nochy D, et al. Predictive power of the second biopsy in lupus nephritis: significance of macrophages. Kidney Int 59:304–316, 2001.
83. Ward MM. Cardiovascular and cerebrovascular morbidity and mortality among women with end-stage renal disease attributable to lupus nephritis. Am J Kidney Dis 36:516–525, 2000.
84. Korbet SM, Lewis EJ, Schwartz MM, Reichlin M, Evans J, Rohde RD. Factors predictive of outcome in severe lupus nephritis. Am J Kidney Dis 35:904–914, 2000.
85. Bono L, Cameron JS, Hicks JA. The very long-term prognosis and complications of lupus nephritis and its treatment. Q J Med 92:211–218, 1999.
86. Adu D, Cross J, Jayne DR. Treatment of systemic lupus erythematosus with mycophenolate mofetil. Lupus 10:203–208, 2001.
87. Sato EI. Methotrexate therapy in systemic lupus erythematosus. Lupus 10:162–164, 2001.
88. Abu-Shakra M, Shoenfeld Y. Azathioprine therapy for patients with systemic lupus erythematosus. Lupus 10:152–153, 2001.
89. Zimmerman R, Radhakrishnan J, Valeri A, Appel G. Advances in the treatment of lupus nephritis. Annu Rev Med 52:63–78, 2001.
90. Ward MM. Changes in the incidence of end-stage renal disease due to lupus nephritis, 1982–1995. Arch Intern Med 160:3136–3140, 2000.
91. Austin HA, Balow JE. Treatment of lupus nephritis. Semin Nephrol 20:265–276, 2000.

92. Boumpas DT, Furie R, Manzi S, et al. A short course of BG9588 (anti-CD40 ligand antibody) improves serologic activity and decreases hematuria in patients with proliferative lupus glomerulonephritis. Arthritis Rheum 48:719–727, 2003.
93. Hebert LA. Management of lupus nephropathy. Nephron 93:C7–C12, 2003.
94. Wang LC, Yang YH, Lu MY, Chiang BL. Retrospective analysis of mortality and morbidity of pediatric systemic lupus erythematosus in the past two decades. J Microbiol Immunol Infect 36:203–208, 2003.
95. Ioannidis JPA, Boki KA, Katsorida ME, et al. Remission, relapse, and re-remission of proliferative lupus nephritis treated with cyclophosphamide. Kidney Int 57:258–264, 2000.
96. Contreras G, Roth D, Pardo V, Striker LG, Schultz DR. Lupus nephritis: a clinical review for practicing nephrologists. Clin Nephrol 57:95–107, 2002.
97. Mok CC, Lai KN. Mycophenolate mofetil in lupus glomerulonephritis. Am J Kidney Dis 40:447–457, 2002.
98. Contreras G, Pardo V, Leclerq B, et al. Sequential therapies for proliferative lupus nephritis. N Engl J Med 350:971–980, 2004.
99. Balow JE, Austin HA III. Treatment of proliferative lupus nephritis. N Engl J Med 43:383–385, 2004.
100. Krane NK, Burjak K, Archie M, O'Donovan R. Persistent lupus activity in end-stage renal disease. Am J Kidney Dis 33:872–879, 1999.

9
Crescentic Glomerulonephritis and Vasculitis

J. CHARLES JENNETTE

Introduction/Clinical Setting

Crescentic glomerulonephritis is not a specific disease but rather is a manifestation of severe glomerular injury that can be caused by many different etiologies and pathogenic mechanisms. The major immunopathologic categories of crescentic glomerulonephritis are immune complex–mediated, anti–glomerular basement membrane (anti-GBM) antibody-mediated, and pauci-immune, which usually is antineutrophil cytoplasmic autoantibody (ANCA)-mediated (1). Table 9.1 shows the relative frequency of these immunopathologic categories of crescentic glomerulonephritis. Crescentic glomerulonephritis can occur as a renal limited process or as a component of systemic small vessel vasculitis, such as Henoch-Schönlein purpura, Goodpasture's syndrome, or ANCA vasculitis (2,3). In addition to small-vessel vasculitis, the kidneys also are a frequent site of involvement by other forms of vasculitis, such as polyarteritis nodosa, Kawasaki disease, giant cell arteritis, and Takayasu arteritis (3).

Anti–Glomerular Basement Membrane Disease

Anti-GBM disease is essentially a small-vessel vasculitis that affects the glomerular capillaries and pulmonary alveolar capillaries (4). It may occur as an isolated glomerulonephritis or as the renal component of a pulmonary-renal syndrome. In the latter instance, the term *Goodpasture's syndrome* is appropriate.

Pathologic Findings

Light Microscopy

By light microscopy, the acute glomerular lesion is characterized by segmental to global fibrinoid necrosis with crescent formation in over 90% of

TABLE 9.1. Frequency of immunopathologic categories of crescentic glomerulonephritis in over 3000 consecutive native kidney biopsies evaluated by immunofluorescence microscopy in the University of North Carolina Nephropathology Laboratory

	Any crescents (n = 487)	>50% crescents (n = 195)	Arteritis in biopsy (n = 37)
Immunohistology			
Pauciimmune (<2+ Ig)	47% (227/487)	61% (118/195)[a]	84% (31/37)
Immune complex (>2+ Ig)	49% (238/487)	29% (56/195)	14% (5/37)[c]
Anti-GBM	5% (25/487)[b]	11% (21/195)	3% (1/37)[d]

[a] 70 of 77 patients tested for ANCA were positive (91%) (44 P-ANCA and 26 C-ANCA).
[b] 3 of 19 patients tested for ANCA were positive (16%) (2 P-ANCA and 1 C-ANCA).
[c] 4 patients had lupus and 1 post-streptococcal glomerulonephritis.
[d] This patient also had a P-ANCA (MPO-ANCA).
From Jennette and Falk (3).

patients (1). Periodic acid-schiff (PAS) and silver stains demonstrate breaks in the GBM in areas of necrosis (Fig. 9.1). Glomerular segments that do not have necrosis often are remarkably normal or have a slight increase in neutrophils. Marked neutrophil infiltration is observed in association with the necrosis in occasional specimens. Features of aggressive immune complex glomerulonephritis are notably absent, such as marked capillary wall thickening and endocapillary hypercellularity. Often there are breaks

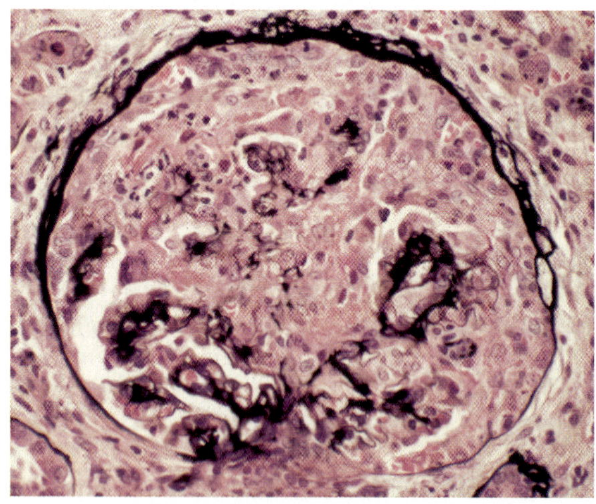

FIGURE 9.1. Glomerulus from a patient with anti–glomerular basement membrane (GBM) disease showing a very large cellular crescent and extensive destruction of approximately 80% of the tuft. A few silver-positive intact profiles of GBM are present at the hilum (Jones silver stain).

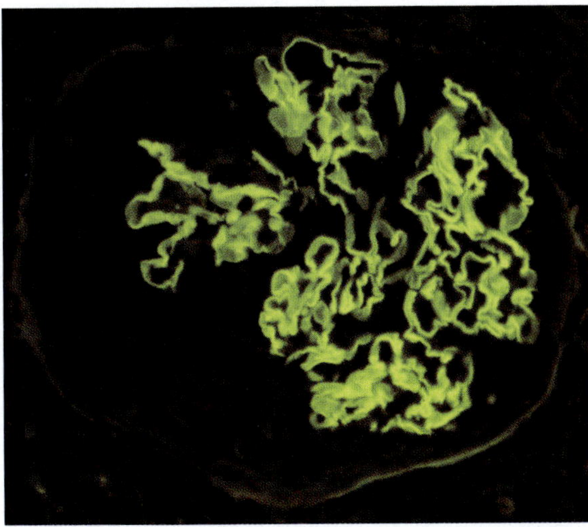

FIGURE 9.2. Glomerulus from a patient with anti-GBM disease showing linear staining of the GBM by direct immunofluorescence microscopy using an antibody specific for immunoglobulin G (IgG).

in Bowman's capsule, occasionally with associated reactive multinucleated giant cells (5).

With time, foci of glomerular necrosis evolve into glomerular sclerosis, and cellular crescents become fibrous crescents. Acute tubulointerstitial inflammation that is centered on necrotic glomeruli evolves to more regional or generalized interstitial fibrosis with chronic inflammation and tubular atrophy.

Immunofluorescence Microscopy

Immunohistology demonstrates intense linear staining of the GBM (Fig. 9.2), predominantly for immunoglobulin G (IgG) along with more granular and discontinuous staining for C3 (Fig. 9.3). Immunoglobulin A (IgA)-dominant anti-GBM disease is very rare (6). Irregular staining for fibrin occurs at sites of fibrinoid necrosis and within crescents. In some specimens, the fibrinoid of glomeruli is so extensive that identification of linear staining along intact segments of GBM is difficult. Care must be taken not to misinterpret anti-GBM disease with extensive destruction of GBMs as pauci-immune disease.

Electron Microscopy

Electron microscopy reveals no immune complex-type electron dense deposits unless there is concurrent immune complex glomerulonephritis.

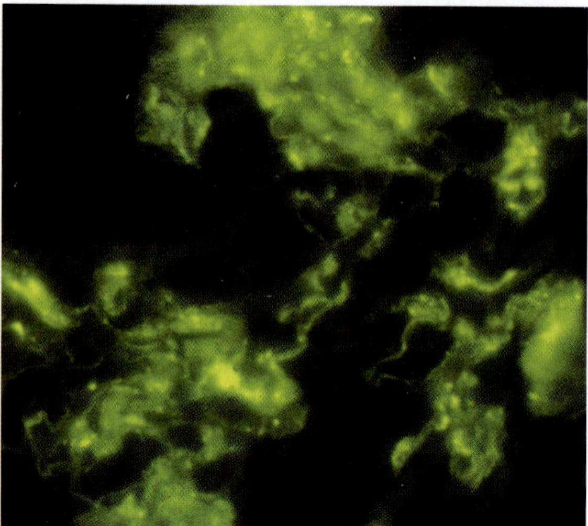

FIGURE 9.3. Glomerulus from a patient with anti-GBM disease showing irregular granular staining of the capillary walls by direct immunofluorescence microscopy using an antibody specific for C3.

Glomerular basement membrane gaps are present in areas of necrosis and crescent formation. Cellular crescents typically contain electron-dense fibrin tactoid strands.

Clinicopathologic Correlations

Anti-GBM disease is caused by autoantibodies directed against the α3 chain in the noncollagenous domain of type 4 collagen (7). Serologic confirmation of anti-GBM disease should be sought, but approximately 10% to 15% of patients with anti-GBM disease have negative results. About a quarter to a third of patients with anti-GBM disease also have ANCA (8). Thus, all anti-GBM patients should be tested for ANCA. Patients with both anti-GBM and ANCA have an intermediate prognosis that is worse than ANCA alone but better than anti-GBM alone. Anti-GBM antibodies characteristically occur as one episode that clears with immunosuppressive therapy, whereas ANCA disease is characterized by more persistent antibodies and frequent recurrence of disease. Patients with combined disease may have permanent remission of the anti-GBM disease with recurrence of the ANCA disease alone.

Approximately half the patients with anti-GBM disease present with rapidly progressive glomerulonephritis without pulmonary hemorrhage and the other half have pulmonary-renal syndrome (Goodpasture's syndrome). However, most patients with pulmonary-renal syndrome have ANCA disease rather than anti-GBM disease (9).

Anti-GBM is the most aggressive form of crescentic glomerulonephritis and has the worst prognosis, especially if aggressive immunosuppressive treatment is not instituted quickly before the serum creatinine is >6 mg/dL (1,10). The serum creatinine at the time treatment is begun is a better predictor of outcome than any pathologic feature. The current approach to treatment uses high-dose cytotoxic agents combined with plasma exchange (10).

Pauci-Immune and ANCA Glomerulonephritis and Vasculitis

Introduction/Clinical Setting

Antineutrophil cytoplasmic autoantibody disease is a form of small-vessel vasculitis (2,3). Small-vessel vasculitides have a predilection for capillaries, venules, and arterioles, although some may affect arteries (2). The major immunopathologic categories of small-vessel vasculitis are anti-GBM disease, immune complex small-vessel vasculitis, and pauci-immune small-vessel vasculitis. Pauci-immune small-vessel vasculitis is characterized by an absence or paucity of vessel staining for immunoglobulin, which is distinct from the conspicuous linear staining in anti-GBM disease and granular staining in immune complex disease. Approximately 85% of active untreated pauci-immune crescentic glomerulonephritis and vasculitis is associated with ANCA in the circulation. The major clinicopathologic expressions of pauci-immune and ANCA-associated vasculitis are (1) renal limited vasculitis (pauci-immune necrotizing and crescentic glomerulonephritis), (2) microscopic polyangiitis, (3) Wegener's granulomatosis, and (4) Churg-Strauss syndrome (Table 9.2) (2,3,11).

Pathologic Findings

Light Microscopy, Immunofluorescence, and Electron Microscopy

Histologically, the glomerular lesion in all four clinicopathologic categories is identical and is characterized by fibrinoid necrosis and crescent formation (Figs. 9.4 to 9.6). In less than 10% of specimens, the glomerulonephritis may be accompanied by necrotizing arteritis (Fig. 9.7) (usually in the interlobular arteries) or medullary angiitis affecting the vasa rectae (Fig. 9.8).

By light microscopy and electron microscopy, pauci-immune crescentic glomerulonephritis cannot be distinguished from anti-GBM crescentic glomerulonephritis; however, immunofluorescence microscopy readily distinguishes the two. Pauci-immune crescentic glomerulonephritis, by definition, has no or low-intensity immunostaining for immunoglobulin; however, often there is some staining for immunoglobulin (12). A reasonable

TABLE 9.2. Names and definitions of vasculitis adopted by the Chapel Hill Consensus Conference on the Nomenclature of Systemic Vasculitis

Large-vessel vasculitis	
Giant cell arteritis	Granulomatous arteritis of the aorta and its major branches, with a predilection for the extracranial branches of the carotid artery. *Often involves the temporal artery. Usually occurs in patients older than 50 and often is associated with polymyalgia rheumatica.*
Takayasu arteritis	Granulomatous inflammation of the aorta and its major branches. *Usually occurs in patients younger than 50.*
Medium-sized vessel vasculitis	
Polyarteritis nodosa	Necrotizing inflammation of medium-sized or small arteries[a] without glomerulonephritis or vasculitis in arterioles, capillaries or venules.
Kawasaki disease	Arteritis involving large, medium-sized, and small arteries, and associated with mucocutaneous lymph node syndrome. *Coronary arteries are often involved. Aorta and veins may be involved. Usually occurs in children.*
Small-vessel vasculitis	
Wegener's granulomatosis	Granulomatous inflammation involving the respiratory tract, and necrotizing vasculitis affecting small to medium-sized vessels, e.g., capillaries, venules, arterioles, and arteries. *Necrotizing glomerulonephritis is common.*
Churg-Strauss syndrome	Eosinophil-rich and granulomatous inflammation involving the respiratory tract and necrotizing vasculitis affecting small to medium-sized vessels, and associated with asthma and blood eosinophilia.
Microscopic polyangiitis	Necrotizing vasculitis with few or no immune deposits affecting small vessels, i.e., capillaries, venules, or arterioles. *Necrotizing arteritis involving small and medium-sized arteries may be present. Necrotizing glomerulonephritis is very common. Pulmonary capillaritis often occurs.*
Henoch-Schönlein purpura	Vasculitis with IgA-dominant immune deposits affecting small vessels, i.e., capillaries, venules, or arterioles. *Typically involves skin, gut and glomeruli, and is associated with arthralgias or arthritis.*
Cryoglobulinemic vasculitis	Vasculitis with cryoglobulin immune deposits affecting small vessels, i.e., capillaries, venules, or arterioles, and associated with cryoglobulins in serum. *Skin and glomeruli are often involved.*

[a] Large artery refers to the aorta and the largest branches directed toward major body regions (e.g., to the extremities and the head and neck); medium-sized artery refers to the main visceral arteries (e.g., renal, hepatic, coronary, and mesenteric arteries), and small artery refers to the distal arterial radicals that connect with arterioles (e.g., renal interlobular arteries). Note that some small and large vessel vasculitides may involve medium-sized arteries, but large and medium-sized vessel vasculitides do not involve vessels smaller than arteries.

Modified from Jennette et al. (11), with permission.

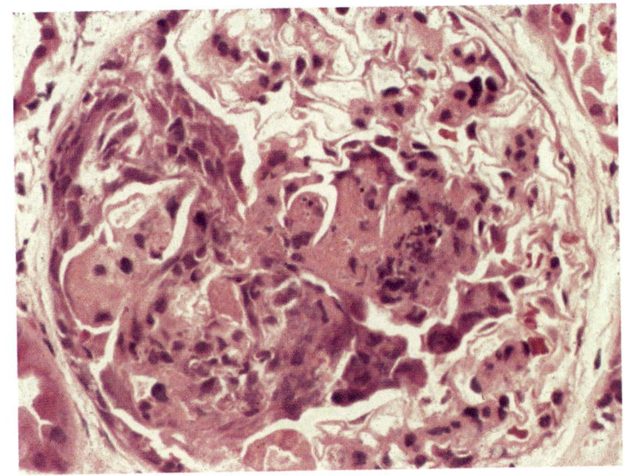

FIGURE 9.4. Glomerulus from a patient with Wegener's granulomatosis demonstrating segmental fibrinoid necrosis and early cellular crescent formation (H&E).

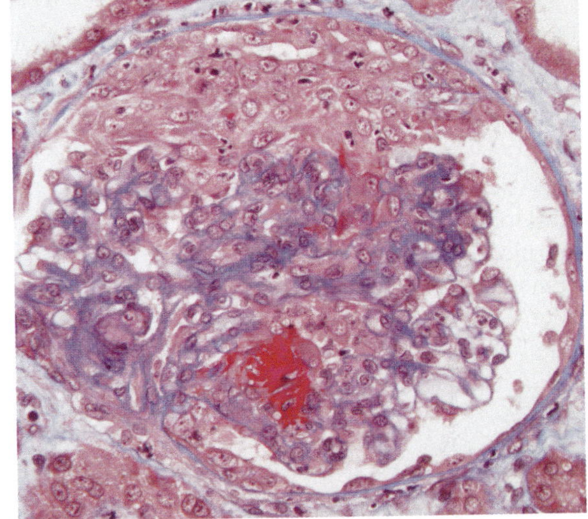

FIGURE 9.5. Glomerulus from a patient with microscopic polyangiitis demonstrating a cellular crescent at the top of the image and a small irregular fuchsinophilic (red) focus of fibrinoid necrosis near the bottom of the image (Masson trichrome stain).

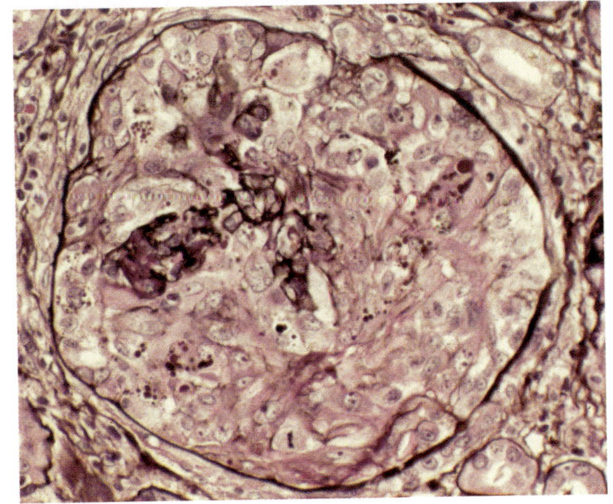

FIGURE 9.6. Glomerulus from a patient with ANCA-positive renal-limited disease showing a large cellular crescent with extensive destruction of the glomerular tuft (Jones silver stain).

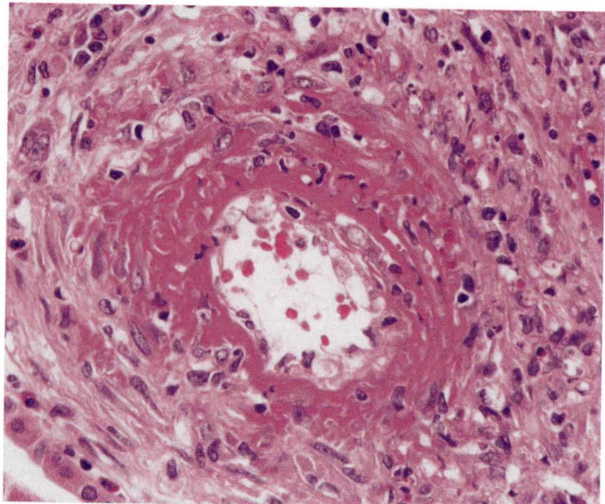

FIGURE 9.7. Interlobular artery in a renal biopsy from a patient with microscopic polyangiitis showing circumferential fibrinoid necrosis with associated leukocyte infiltration and leukocytoclasia (H&E).

approach is to draw the line at 2+ or less immunoglobulin staining on a scale of 0 to 4+ for pauci-immune disease. Pauci-immune crescentic glomerulonephritis often has irregular segmental or global staining for fibrin at sites of fibrinoid necrosis and crescent formation (Fig. 9.9). Electron microscopy may show no electron-dense deposits, or there may be a few small electron-dense deposits, especially if immunofluorescence micros-

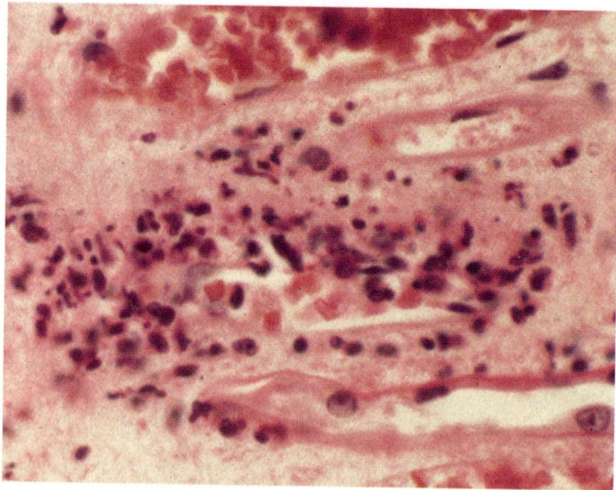

FIGURE 9.8. Medullary vasa recta in a renal biopsy from a patient with Wegener's granulomatosis showing angiitis with leukocytoclasia (H&E).

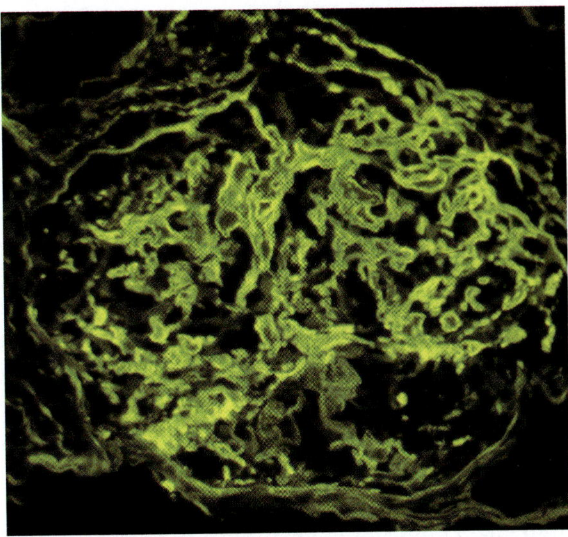

FIGURE 9.9. Glomerulus from a patient with ANCA crescentic glomerulonephritis irregular staining of a large crescent by direct immunofluorescence microscopy using an antibody specific for fibrin.

copy revealed staining for immunoglobulin. Glomerular basement membrane breaks often can be identified.

Microscopic polyangiitis is necrotizing vasculitis with few or no immune deposits affecting small vessels, that is, capillaries, venules, or arterioles (11,13). Necrotizing arteritis occurs in some but not all patients. Approximately 90% of patients with microscopic polyangiitis have glomerulonephritis. Hemorrhagic pulmonary alveolar capillaritis is common in patients with microscopic polyangiitis. Histologically, the acute vascular lesions, for example, affecting dermal venules or small visceral arteries, are characterized by segmental fibrinoid necrosis, and mural and perivascular neutrophilic infiltration with leukocytoclasia (Figs. 9.7 and 9.8). Within a few days, the predominant inflammatory cells in the vasculitic lesions evolve from neutrophils to mononuclear leukocytes, and the fibrinoid necrosis transforms into fibrosis.

Wegener's granulomatosis is characterized by granulomatous inflammation that frequently is accompanied by necrotizing vasculitis affecting capillaries, venules, arterioles, and small to medium-sized arteries (11). Necrotizing granulomatous inflammation is observed most often in the upper and lower respiratory tract, but occasionally in other tissues, such as the orbit, skin, and kidneys. The granulomatous lesions typically have extensive necrosis with infiltrating mononuclear and polymorphonuclear leukocytes with scattered multinucleated giant cells. Necrotizing glomerulonephritis is common (Fig. 9.4). The vasculitis in the lungs and elsewhere can involve arteries, arterioles, veins, venules, and capillaries, and can be granulomatous or nongranulomatous. The latter is histologically identical to the necrotizing vasculitis of microscopic polyangiitis and Churg-Strauss syndrome.

Churg-Strauss syndrome is characterized by eosinophil-rich granulomatous inflammation involving the respiratory tract and necrotizing vasculitis affecting small to medium-sized vessels that is associated with asthma and blood eosinophilia (11). The vasculitis of Churg-Strauss syndrome cannot be definitively differentiated by histology from the vasculitis of Wegener's granulomatosis or microscopic polyangiitis; however, there is a tendency for more eosinophils among the infiltrating leukocytes. Likewise, the necrotizing granulomatous inflammation of Churg-Strauss syndrome resembles that of Wegener's granulomatosis but tends to have more eosinophils. The vasculitis of Churg-Strauss syndrome most often affects the lungs, heart, peripheral nervous system, skin, gut, and kidneys. The pauci-immune focal necrotizing glomerulonephritis of Churg-Strauss syndrome usually is less severe than the glomerulonephritis in Wegener's granulomatosis or microscopic polyangiitis, but is histologically indistinguishable.

Etiology/Pathogenesis

Overall, approximately 85% of patients with pauci-immune crescentic glomerulonephritis or pauci-immune small-vessel vasculitis have circulating ANCA. The two major antigen specificities of ANCA are for proteinase 3 (PR3-ANCA) or myeloperoxidase (MPO-ANCA). Either specificity can occur in any clinicopathologic variant of ANCA-disease, but MPO-ANCA is most prevalent in renal-limited disease and PR3-ANCA is most prevalent in Wegener's granulomatosis.

There is compelling in vitro (14) and animal model (15,16) experimental data showing that ANCA IgG causes glomerulonephritis and vasculitis, probably by direct interaction with neutrophils (and possibly monocytes) resulting in activation with release of lytic enzymes and reactive oxygen radicals that cause the inflammatory injury to glomeruli and vessels. Strong clinical support is provided by the observation that a neonate developed pulmonary hemorrhage and nephritis following transplacental transfer of maternal MPO-ANCA IgG (17).

Clinicopathologic Correlations

All variants of pauci-immune small-vessel vasculitis and glomerulonephritis are treated with high-dose corticosteroids and immunosuppressive agents when there is active and progressive glomerulonephritis (18,19). Remission of glomerulonephritis and other vasculitic manifestations can be induced in approximately 80% of patients. However, a third or more of patients may have one of more relapses within 5 years. Nevertheless, the

5-year renal and patient survival approaches 80% if treatment is instituted early enough. As with anti-GBM disease, the renal outcome in ANCA disease correlates best with the serum creatinine at the time treatment was begun. In one study, the pathologic finding that correlated best with outcome was the percentage of normal-appearing glomeruli by light microscopy (20).

Polyarteritis Nodosa

Introduction/Clinical Setting

Polyarteritis is categorized as a medium-sized vessel vasculitides because it primarily affects medium-sized arteries rather than smaller vessels (11). The other major category of medium-sized vessel vasculitis is Kawasaki disease (Table 9.2). Medium-sized vessel vasculitides have a predilection for main visceral arteries, such as the coronary, hepatic, renal, and mesenteric arteries and their major first- and second-order branches. These same vessels, however, also can be involved with large-vessel vasculitides and small-vessel vasculitides. In the kidney, the major targets of polyarteritis nodosa and Kawasaki disease are the interlobar and arcuate arteries, whereas ANCA small-vessel vasculitis primarily targets interlobular arteries, arterioles, vasa rectae, and glomerular capillaries (3).

The term *polyarteritis nodosa* has been used quite variably over the years (2). Some definitions have allowed involvement of vessels smaller than arteries, including glomerulonephritis. However, the Chapel Hill nomenclature system confined the term to necrotizing arteritis that affects arteries but does not involve vessels smaller than arteries, and thus does not cause glomerulonephritis (11). If pauci-immune necrotizing arteritis is associated with glomerulonephritis, this would be categorized as microscopic polyangiitis by the Chapel Hill nomenclature system.

Pathologic Findings

Light Microscopy

By light microscopy, polyarteritis nodosa is characterized by segmental transmural fibrinoid necrosis and accompanying inflammation (Fig. 9.10), which initially has predominantly neutrophils and sometimes eosinophils, but within several days has predominantly mononuclear leukocytes. The segmental inflammation and necrosis in artery walls may produce an aneurysm (actually a pseudoaneurysm) by eroding through the artery wall into the perivascular tissue. Infarction and hemorrhage are the major consequences of renal involvement by polyarteritis nodosa.

Polyarteritis nodosa is treated with high-dose corticosteroids, often in combination with cytotoxic drugs such as cyclophosphamide (21). Polyar-

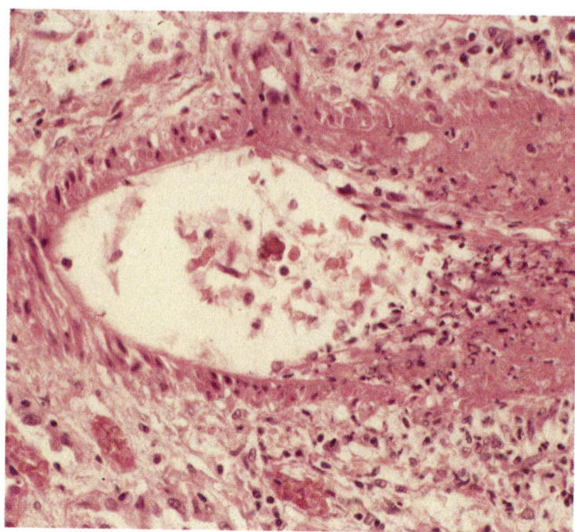

FIGURE 9.10. Arcuate artery in a renal biopsy from a patient with polyarteritis nodosa showing segmental fibrinoid necrosis with associated leukocyte infiltration and leukocytoclasia (H&E).

teritis nodosa is less likely to recur after induction of remission than is microscopic polyangiitis.

Kawasaki Disease

The sine qua non of Kawasaki disease is the mucocutaneous lymph node syndrome, which includes fever, cutaneous, and oral mucosal erythema and sloughing, and lymphadenopathy (11,22). Kawasaki disease is a disease of childhood that rarely occurs after the age of 5 years. The vasculitic lesions of Kawasaki disease involve predominantly small and medium-sized arteries, with a special predilection for the coronary arteries (22). The histologic lesions are characterized by segmental transmural edema and necrosis with infiltration by monocytes and neutrophils (Fig. 9.11). The necrotizing lesions of Kawasaki disease have less fibrinoid material and more edema than the necrotizing lesions of polyarteritis nodosa.

Kawasaki disease rarely causes clinically significant renal disease; however, postmortem examination demonstrates substantial involvement of renal arteritis in many patients who die from Kawasaki disease (22).

The arteritis of Kawasaki disease respond very well to treatment with aspirin and high-dose intravenous immunoglobulin (23).

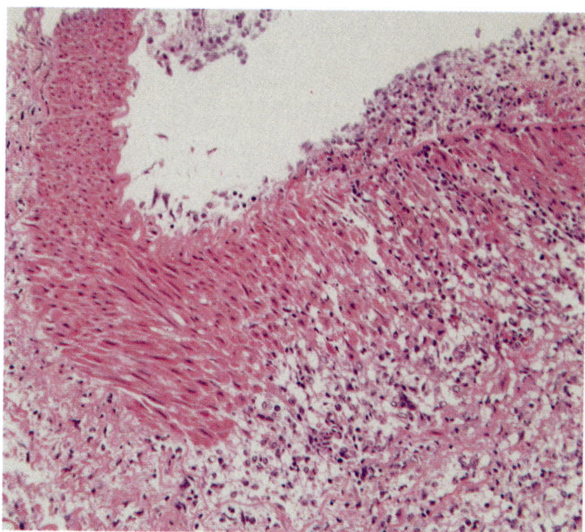

FIGURE 9.11. Lobar artery in a postmortem kidney specimen from a patient with Kawasaki disease showing segmental necrosis with associated edema and leukocyte infiltration (H&E).

Large-Vessel Vasculitis

Introduction/Clinical Setting

Large-vessel vasculitis affects the aorta and its major branches with transmural chronic inflammation that is characterized even in the acute phase by infiltration of predominantly mononuclear leukocytes, often with accompanying multinucleated giant cells (11). The two major clinicopathologic variants are giant cell arteritis and Takayasu arteritis. The best distinguishing feature between these two variants is the age of the patient (11). Giant cell arteritis rarely occurs before 50 years of age and Takayasu arteritis virtually always occurs prior to the age of 50. Postmortem examination reveals that pathologic involvement of the kidneys by large-vessel vasculitis is much more common than clinically significant involvement (3). The most common clinical manifestation is renovascular hypertension, which results form involvement of the main renal artery or its major branches, especially the lobar (interlobar) arteries (24,25).

Pathologic Findings

The pathologic hallmark of large-vessel vasculitis is transmural infiltration of artery walls by mononuclear leukocytes accompanied by variable numbers of multinucleated giant cells (Fig. 9.12). This often results in

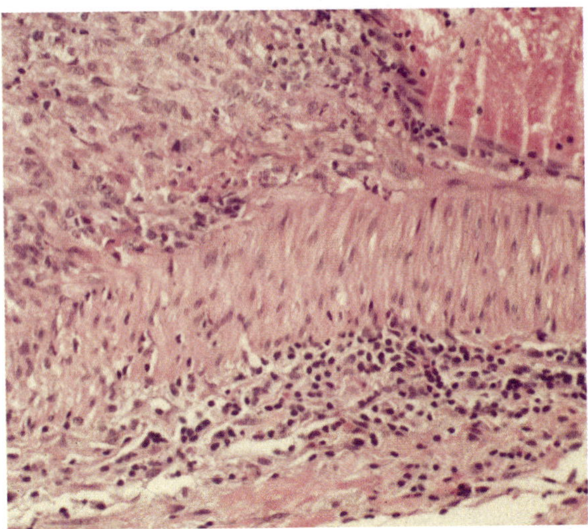

FIGURE 9.12. Renal artery in a nephrectomy specimen from a patient with giant cell arteritis showing (on the left) transmural inflammation with a markedly thickened intima that is impinging on the lumen (H&E).

thickening of the intima and narrowing of the lumen, which causes ischemia to the tissue supplied by the artery. Involvement of the renal artery can cause a pattern of renal artery stenosis atrophy in the renal parenchyma that is characterized by marked reduction in the size of the tubules and resultant clustering of glomeruli close to one another. This pattern of atrophy has much less interstitial fibrosis and inflammation than the ischemic atrophy of hypertensive arterionephrosclerosis.

Large-vessel vasculitis that is causing substantial ischemic injury is treated with corticosteroids (24,25). Surgical revascularization may be required if corticosteroids are not adequate to prevent important end-organ damage.

References

1. Jennette JC. Rapidly progressive and crescentic glomerulonephritis. Kidney Int 63:1164–1172, 2003.
2. Jennette JC, Falk RJ. Small vessel vasculitis. N Engl J Med 337:1512–1523, 1997.
3. Jennette JC, Falk RJ. The pathology of vasculitis involving the kidney. Am J Kidney Dis 24:130–141, 1994.
4. Savage CO, Pusey CD, Bowman C, Rees AJ, Lockwood CM. Antiglomerular basement membrane antibody mediated disease in the British Isles 1980–4. Br Med J Clin Res Ed 292:301–304, 1986.

5. Bajema IM, Hagen EC, Ferrario F, et al. Renal granulomas in systemic vasculitis. EC/BCR Project for ANCA-Assay Standardization. Clin Nephrol 48:16–21, 1997.
6. Borza DB, Chedid MF, Colon S, Lager DJ, Leung N, Fervenza FC. Recurrent Goodpasture's disease secondary to a monoclonal IgA1-kappa antibody autoreactive with the alpha1/alpha2 chains of type IV collagen. Am J Kidney Dis 45:397–406, 2005.
7. Hellmark T, Johansson C, Wieslander J. Characterization of anti-GBM antibodies involved in Goodpasture's syndrome. Kidney Int 46:823–829, 1994.
8. Short AK, Esnault VL, Lockwood CM. Anti-neutrophil cytoplasm antibodies and anti-glomerular basement membrane antibodies: two coexisting distinct autoreactivities detectable in patients with rapidly progressive glomerulonephritis. Am J Kidney Dis 26:439–445, 1995.
9. Niles JL, Bottinger EP, Saurina GR, et al. The syndrome of lung hemorrhage and nephritis is usually an ANCA-associated condition. Arch Intern Med 56:440–445, 1996.
10. Levy JB, Turner AN, Rees AJ, Pusey CD. Long-term outcome of anti-glomerular basement membrane antibody disease treated with plasma exchange and immunosuppression. Ann Intern Med 134:1033–1042, 2001.
11. Jennette JC, Falk RJ, Andrassy K, et al. Nomenclature of systemic vasculitides. Proposal of an international consensus conference. Arthritis Rheum 37:187–192, 1994.
12. Harris AA, Falk RJ, Jennette JC. Crescentic glomerulonephritis with a paucity of glomerular immunoglobulin localization. Am J Kidney Dis 32:179–184, 1998.
13. Jennette JC, Thomas DB, Falk RJ. Microscopic polyangiitis (microscopic polyarteritis). Semin Diagn Pathol 18:3–13, 2001.
14. Jennette JC, Falk RJ. Pathogenesis of the vascular and glomerular damage in ANCA-positive vasculitis. Nephrol Dial Transplant 13 (suppl) 1:16–20, 1998.
15. Xiao H, Heeringa P, Hu P, et al. Antineutrophil cytoplasmic autoantibodies specific for myeloperoxidase cause glomerulonephritis and vasculitis in mice. J Clin Invest 110:955–963, 2002.
16. Xiao H, Heeringa P, Liu Z, et al. A major role for neutrophils in anti-myeloperoxidase antibody induced necrotizing and crescentic glomerulonephritis. Am J Pathol 167:39–45, 2005.
17. Bansal PJ, Tobin MC. Neonatal microscopic polyangiitis secondary to transfer of maternal myeloperoxidase-antineutrophil cytoplasmic antibody resulting in neonatal pulmonary hemorrhage and renal involvement. Ann Allergy Asthma Immunol 93:398–401, 2004.
18. Bacon PA. Therapy of vasculitis. J Rheumatol 21:788–790, 1994.
19. Nachman PH, Hogan SL, Jennette JC, Falk RJ. Treatment response and relapse in ANCA-associated microscopic polyangiitis and glomerulonephritis. J Am Soc Nephrol 7:33–39, 1996.
20. Bajema IM, Hagen EC, Ferrario F, et al. Renal granulomas in systemic vasculitis. EC/BCR Project for ANCA-Assay Standardization. Clin Nephrol 48:16–21, 1997.
21. Guillevin L, Lhote F. Treatment of polyarteritis nodosa and microscopic polyangiitis. Arthritis Rheum 41:2100–2105, 1998.

22. Naoe S, Takahashi K, Masuda H, Tanaka N. Kawasaki disease. With particular emphasis on arterial lesions. Acta Pathol Jpn 41:785–797, 1991.
23. Newburger JW, Takahashi M, Burns JC, et al. The treatment of Kawasaki syndrome with intravenous gamma globulin. N Engl J Med 315:341–347, 1986.
24. Sonnenblick M, Nasher G, Rosin A. Nonclassical organ involvement in temporal arteritis. Semin Arthritis Rheum 19:183–190, 1989.
25. Lagneau P, Michel JB. Renovascular hypertension and Takayasu's disease. J Urol 134:876–879, 1985.

Section V
Vascular Diseases

10
Nephrosclerosis and Hypertension

AGNES B. FOGO

Arterionephrosclerosis

Introduction/Clinical Setting

Approximately 60 million people in the United States have hypertension. Many are undiagnosed or untreated. Different populations have different risks and different consequences of hypertension. Increased hypertension is seen with aging, positive family history, African-American race, and exogenous factors such as smoking. Although African Americans make up only 12% of the U.S. population, they are fivefold overrepresented among patients with end-stage renal disease (ESRD) presumed due to hypertension (1,2). Hypertension is associated with significant morbidity and mortality due both to cardiovascular and renal diseases (1–5).

Essential hypertension is diagnosed when no cause is found. Hypertension may also be secondary to various hormonal abnormalities, including excess aldosterone, norepinephrine, or epinephrine, or produced from adrenal cortical, medullary, or other tumors, renin-producing tumors, or hypercalcemia or hyperparathyroidism. Other secondary causes include neurogenic, iatrogenic, and structural lesions (e.g., coarctation of the aorta).

Renal hypertension refers to hypertension secondary to renal disease. Chronic renal disease is the most common form of secondary hypertension (5–6% of all hypertension). The kidneys modulate blood pressure in several ways: They modulate salt/water balance under the influence of *aldosterone*. The kidney is also a major site of renin production, which allows generation of *angiotensin II*, an important vasoconstrictor and stimulus for aldosterone secretion. In renovascular disease (i.e., stenosis of the renal artery), renal ischemia is thought to be the stimulus that increases renin-angiotensin system activity, thereby increasing systemic blood pressure. In renal parenchymal disease, multiple factors contribute to increased blood pressure. The decreased mass of functioning nephrons leads to a decrease in the glomerular filtration rate (GFR), leading to increased extracellular volume, increased angiotensin, aldosterone, and other vasoactive substances.

The most common complications in untreated hypertension are cardiac, renal, and retinal disease. Half of hypertensive patients die of cardiac disease, 10% to 15% of cerebrovascular disease, and about 10% of renal failure. Treatment to decrease blood pressure reduces mortality, and especially reduces the incidence of cerebrovascular accidents. Hypertension accelerates the decline in GFR characteristic of many chronic renal diseases, whether the primary cause is hypertension associated or not. Chronic renal disease is common, affecting 195,000 Americans, with 45,000 new patients enrolled in end-stage treatment Medicare programs yearly. It has been postulated that direct transmission of increased blood pressure to the glomerulus increases injury. Other mechanisms may also play a role, however, since antihypertensive drugs have benefit even in nonhypertensive patients with chronic renal disease (see below).

Pathologic Findings

Gross Findings/Light Microscopy

"Benign" nephrosclerosis results in small kidneys with finely granular surface and thinned cortex in late stages. Malignant (accelerated) nephrosclerosis grossly shows petechial hemorrhage of the subcapsular surface, with mottling and occasional areas of infarct. Microscopically, in "benign" arterionephrosclerosis there is vascular wall medial thickening with frequent afferent arteriolar hyaline deposits, and varying degree of intimal fibrosis. The hyalinization is due to endothelial injury and increased pressure, leading to an insudate of plasma macromolecules. There are associated focal glomerular ischemic changes with variable thickening and wrinkling of the basement membrane, and/or global sclerosis, tubular atrophy, and interstitial fibrosis (Fig. 10.1). Global sclerosis more commonly is of the obsolescent type, with fibrous material obliterating Bowman's space. Solidified glomeruli, where the tuft is globally sclerosed without collagen in Bowman's space, has been called "decompensated" arterionephrosclerosis. Secondary focal segmental glomerulosclerosis (FSGS) may also occur, often with associated glomerular basement membrane (GBM) corrugation and filling of Bowman's space with fibrous material (4–10). These morphologic features hint that the segmental sclerotic process is secondary to hypertension-associated injury, rather than idiopathic FSGS. The lesions of accelerated hypertension-associated consist of mucoid change of the arterioles, often with red blood cell (RBC) fragments within the wall. In malignant hypertension, arterioles show fibrinoid necrosis, and interlobular arteries have a concentric onion-skin pattern of intimal fibrosis, overlapping with the appearance of progressive systemic sclerosis

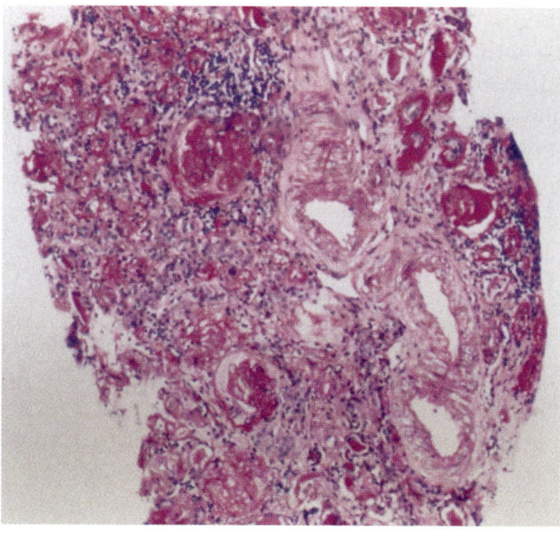

FIGURE 10.1. Arterial and arteriolar medial thickening, intimal and interstitial fibrosis, tubular atrophy and global sclerosis in arterionephrosclerosis (PAS).

and thrombotic microangiopathy (Fig. 10.2) (see below). There is proportional tubulointerstitial fibrosis in arterionephrosclerosis.

Immunofluorescence may show trapping of IgM and C3 in glomeruli, but there are no immune complex–type deposits. In malignant hypertension, fibrin/fibrinogen staining may be present in necrosed arterioles/arteries and injured glomeruli.

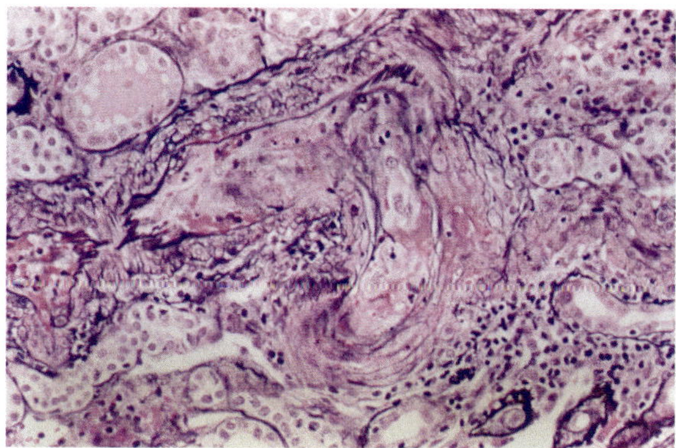

FIGURE 10.2. Vascular fibrinoid necrosis and thrombosis in malignant hypertension (Jones silver stain).

Electron microscopy confirms the corrugated, wrinkled GBM, and ischemic changes with increased lamina rara interna but without immune deposits. Hyaline may be present in sclerosed segments. Some foot process effacement may also be present, but it is usually not extensive.

Although none of the above lesions is pathognomonic, the constellation of these changes in the absence of other lesions of primary glomerular disease is indicative of arterionephrosclerosis.

Etiology/Pathogenesis

Hypertension has been presumed to cause end-organ damage in the kidney, and hypertension undoubtedly accelerates progressive scarring of renal parenchyma, but the relationship of hypertension and arterionephrosclerosis is not simple and linear (11). In a large series of renal biopsies in patients with essential hypertension, arterionephrosclerosis was present in the vast majority, and the severity of arteriolar sclerosis correlated significantly with level of diastolic blood pressure (9). However, in several large autopsy series of patients with presumed benign hypertension, significant renal lesions were rare (4,5). Further, the level of blood pressure does not directly predict degree of end-organ damage: African-Americans have higher risk for more severe end-organ damage at any level of blood pressure (2). The African American Study of Kidney Disease (AASK) trial showed that African Americans with presumed arterionephrosclerosis indeed did not have other lesions, by renal biopsy, but the global sclerosis was severe and did not correlate with vascular sclerosis (12). It is possible that underlying microvascular disease causes the hypertension and the renal disease in susceptible patients. Underlying causes include possible genetic and structural components, such as decreased nephron number and consequently fewer, but enlarged glomeruli (13). Our data suggest a different phenotype of scarring in hypertensive nephrosclerosis in African Americans vs. Caucasians, with solidified global glomerulosclerosis prevalent in the former, contrasting with the obsolescent type (see above) in Caucasians (14). The AASK trial has shown that angiotensin-converting enzyme inhibitors (ACEIs) are effective in protecting renal function in African Americans, although multiple additional drugs were needed to achieve blood pressure control (15).

Cholesterol Emboli

Introduction/Clinical Setting

Patients with significant atherosclerosis are also at risk for cholesterol embolization due to dislodgment of atheromatous plaque material. These emboli shower organs downstream from the site of origin in the aorta, and

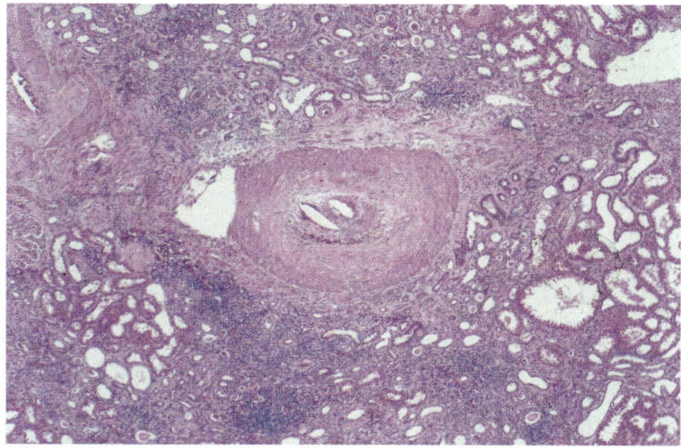

FIGURE 10.3. Cholesterol emboli in artery with surrounding mononuclear and early fibrotic reaction (PAS).

thus often involve the kidney, skin, gastrointestinal (GI) tract, adrenals, pancreas, and testes. Cholesterol emboli may occur spontaneously or after an invasive vascular procedure. This entity mimics vasculitis clinically, and presents with acute renal failure, new-onset or exacerbated hypertension, and eosinophilia (16–18). In some patients, there is associated presumed secondary FSGS, with proteinuria.

Pathologic Findings

Cholesterol crystals usually lodge in and occlude interlobular size arteries (Fig. 10.3). The crystals themselves are dissolved by processing of tissue, but cleft-shaped empty spaces remain, with surrounding mononuclear cell reaction, which over weeks organizes to fibrous tissue. Vessels typically show associated arteriosclerosis, with proportional tubulointerstitial fibrosis and glomerulosclerosis (17–19). The cholesterol emboli are very focally distributed, and serial section analysis may be necessary to detect diagnostic lesions. Immunofluorescence and electron microscopy do not show any specific lesions.

Scleroderma (Progressive Systemic Sclerosis)

Introduction/Clinical Setting

Progressive systemic sclerosis (PSS) is a multisystem disease that affects the skin, the GI tract, the lung, the heart, and the kidney. In the cutaneous limited form (CREST: calcinosis, Raynaud's phenomenon, esophageal hypomotility, sclerodactyly, and telangiectasia), visceral involvement typically takes much longer to become manifest. Kidney involvement is rare in CREST patients, occurring in ~1% (19,20).

In PSS, kidney involvement occurs in approximately 60% to 70%. Scleroderma renal crisis, manifest by malignant hypertension, acute renal failure, some even with infarcts, develops in approximately 20% of patients with PSS (21). Age at onset of systemic sclerosis is 30 to 50 years, and females are affected more than males.

Pathologic Findings

Gross Findings/Light Microscopy

Grossly, petechial hemorrhages or even renal infarcts may be present in patients with scleroderma renal crisis, similar to hemolytic uremic syndrome or malignant hypertension. Microscopically, there is fibrinoid necrosis of afferent arterioles. Interlobular arteries show intimal thickening, proliferation of endothelial cells, and edema. Red blood cell fragments are often present within the injured vessel wall, and there may be vessel wall necrosis and/or fibrin thrombi within vessels. Glomeruli may show ischemic collapse, or fibrinoid necrosis. In chronic injury, arterioles show reduplication of the elastic internal lamina, so-called onion skin pattern (Fig. 10.4). Tubules may show degeneration and even necrosis, especially in scleroderma crisis. Tubulointerstitial fibrosis develops with chronic injury (19,20).

Immunofluorescence Microscopy

There are no immune complexes, although sclerotic segments of glomeruli may show IgM and C3. Necrosed vessels may show fibrin and fibrinogen.

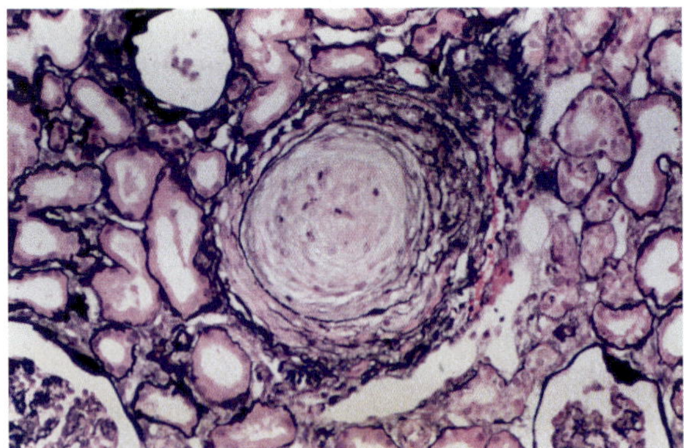

FIGURE 10.4. Onion-skinning appearance in progressive systemic sclerosis with concentric intimal proliferation and fibrosis and mucoid change (Jones silver stain).

Electron Microscopy

There is corrugation of the GBM and increased lucency of the lamina rara interna, without immune deposits.

Thus, the pathologic appearance of PSS overlaps with that of malignant hypertension and thrombotic microangiopathy (TMA). Idiopathic malignant hypertension tends to involve smaller vessels, that is, afferent arterioles, whereas PSS may extend to interlobular size and larger vessels, and TMA typically involves primarily glomeruli. However, distinction of PSS and malignant hypertension solely on morphologic grounds is not feasible, and clinicopathologic correlation is required for specific diagnosis.

Etiology/Pathogenesis

The pathogenesis of PSS is probably immune with unknown inciting events. Autoantibodies are often present, including anti-topoisomerase I, anticentromere, and anti-RNA polymerase, each present in 25%. Only one of these markers may be positive in any one patient. Some studies have demonstrated cytotoxic antiendothelial factors in serum from PSS patients. Imbalance of vasodilators (e.g., nitric oxide, vasodilatory neuropeptides such as calcitonin gene-related peptide, substance P) and vasoconstrictors (e.g., endothelin-1, serotonin, thromboxane A_2) has been described in scleroderma patients. Prolonged vasoconstriction could contribute to structural changes and fibrosis in the kidney as well. Endothelial injury is thought to play a key role in renal PSS, but whether it is primary or initiated by immune injury has not been elucidated. A defect in circulating endothelial progenitor cells in PSS patients has been proposed to underlie deficiency of vasculogenesis and repair in response to endothelial injury, contributing to sclerosis (22).

References

1. Blythe WB, Maddux FW. Hypertension as a causative diagnosis of patients entering end-stage renal disease programs in the United States from 1980 to 1986. Am J Kidney Dis 18:33–37, 1991.
2. Toto RB. Hypertensive nephrosclerosis in African Americans. Kidney Int 64:2331–2341, 2003.
3. Lopes AA, Port FK, James SA, Agodoa L. The excess risk of treated end-stage renal disease in blacks in the United States. J Am Soc Nephrol 3:1961–1971, 1993.
4. Olson JL. Hypertension: essential and secondary forms. In: Heptinstall's Pathology of the Kidney, 5th ed. Jennette JC, Olson JL, Schwartz M, Silva FG, eds. Philadelphia: Lippincott-Raven, 1998:943–1001.
5. Kincaid-Smith P, Whitworth JA. Hypertension and the kidney. In: The Kidney: A Clinicopathologic Study. Eds: Kincaid-Smith P, Whitworth JA. Melbourne: Blackwell, 1987:131.

6. Sommers SC, Relman AS, Smithwick RH. Histologic studies of kidney biopsy specimens from patients with hypertension. Am J Pathol 34:685–713, 1958.
7. Katz SM, Lavin L, Swartz C. Glomerular lesions in benign essential hypertension. Arch Pathol Lab Med 103:199–203, 1979.
8. McManus JFA, Lupton CH Jr. Ischemic obsolescence of renal glomeruli: the natural history of the lesions and their relation to hypertension. Lab Invest 9:413–434, 1960.
9. Bohle A, Wehrmann M, Greschniok A, Junghans R. Renal morphology in essential hypertension: analysis of 1177 unselected cases. Kidney Int Suppl 67: S205–S206, 1998.
10. Böhle A, Ratschek M. The compensated and decompensated form of benign nephrosclerosis. Pathol Res Pract 174:357–367, 1982.
11. Meyrier A, Simon P. Nephroangiosclerosis and hypertension: things are not as simple as you might think. Nephrol Dial Transplant 11:2116–2120, 1996.
12. Fogo A, Breyer JA, Smith MC, et al. Accuracy of the diagnosis of hypertensive nephrosclerosis in African Americans: a report from the African American Study of Kidney Disease (AASK) trial. AASK Pilot Study Investigators. Kidney Int 51:244–252, 1997.
13. Keller G, Zimmer G, Mall G, et al. Nephron number in patients with primary hypertension. N Engl J Med 348:101–108, 2003.
14. Marcantoni C, Ma L-J, Federspiel C, Fogo AB. Hypertensive nephrosclerosis in African-Americans vs Caucasians. Kidney Int 62:172–180, 2002.
15. Agodoa LY, Appel L, Bakris GL, et al. Effect of ramipril vs amlodipine on renal outcomes in hypertensive nephrosclerosis: a randomized controlled trial. JAMA 285:2719–2728, 2001.
16. Fine MJ, Kapoor W, Falanga V. Cholesterol crystal embolization: a review of 221 cases in the English literature. Angiology 38:769–784, 1987.
17. Greenberg A, Bastacky SI, Iqbal A, et al. Focal segmental glomerulosclerosis associated with nephrotic syndrome in cholesterol atheroembolism: clinicopathological correlations. Am J Kidney Dis 29:334–344, 1997.
18. Fogo A, Stone WJ. Atheroembolic renal disease. In: Martinez-Maldonado M, ed. Hypertension and Renal Disease in the Elderly. Cambridge, MA: Blackwell Scientific, 1998:261–271.
19. Leinwand I, Duryee AW, Richter MN. Scleroderma (based on study of over 150 cases). Ann Intern Med 41:1003–1041, 1954.
20. Donohoe JF. Scleroderma and the kidney. Kidney Int 41:462–477, 1992.
21. Steen VD, Medsger TA Jr. Long-term outcomes of scleroderma renal crisis. Ann Intern Med 133:600–603, 2000.
22. Kuwana M, Okazaki Y, Yasuoka H, Kawakami Y, Ikeda Y. Defective vasculogenesis in systemic sclerosis. Lancet 364:603–610, 2004.

11 Thrombotic Microangiopathies

Agnes B. Fogo

Introduction/Clinical Setting

Hemolytic uremic syndrome (HUS) and thrombotic thrombocytopenic purpura (TTP) share the morphologic lesion of thrombotic microangiopathy (TMA), characterized by platelet thrombi occluding the microvasculature. The HUS and TTP syndromes overlap clinically (1–9). Recent evidence indicates differing pathogenesis (see below): TTP is more common in adults, and is characterized by fever, bleeding, hemolytic anemia, renal failure, and neurologic impairment. Hemolytic uremic syndrome is characterized by acute renal failure, nonimmune hemolytic anemia, and thrombocytopenia, and it is most common in infants and small children. The renal manifestations at presentation include hematuria and low-grade proteinuria with elevated creatinine in severe cases. Intravascular hemolysis is evident by increased bilirubin and lactate dehydrogenase (LDH), reticulocytosis, and low haptoglobin. Both HUS and TTP cause thrombocytopenia, but in our experience, and that of others, this may not be detected by the time a renal biopsy is performed, especially in the transplant setting (10).

Pathologic Findings

Light Microscopy

Fibrin and platelet thrombi are present, primarily in the glomeruli (1–4). Fibrin is best visualized on hematoxylin and eosin or silver stains. Lesions may extend to arterioles, with some overlap with progressive malignant hypertension and systemic sclerosis, where arteriolar and even larger vessel involvement occurs (Figs. 11.1 and 11.2). Mesangiolysis occurs frequently, but is a focal, subtle lesion that may be overlooked (11). Mesangial areas seem to "unravel," resulting in very long, sausage-shaped capillary loops due to the loss of mesangial integrity and coalescence of adjoining loops.

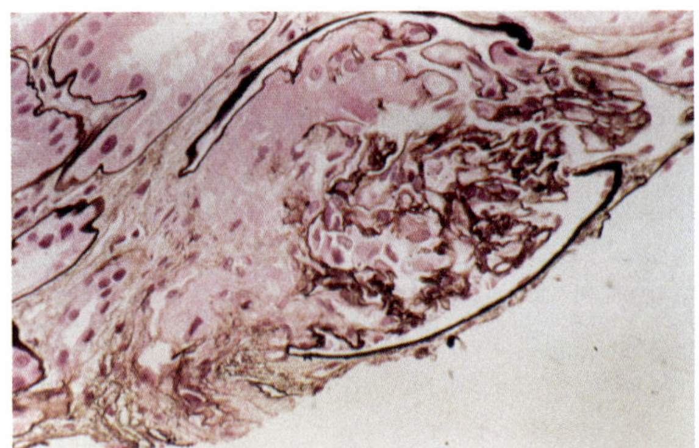

FIGURE 11.1. Segmental red blood cells (RBCs) and fibrin in capillary loops and arteriole in glomerulus in thrombotic microangiopathy (Jones silver stain).

In infants and young children, thrombotic lesions predominate (4). In older children and adults, varied lesions occur. Many glomeruli may show only ischemic changes with corrugation of the glomerular basement membrane and retraction and collapse of the glomerular tuft. Segmental glomerular necrosis may be seen with rare well-developed fibrin thrombi. Arterioles and arteries, when involved, show thrombosis and sometimes necrosis of the vessel wall, with intimal swelling, mucoid change and intimal proliferation. Fragmentation of red blood cells within the vessel wall may also be seen. Tubular and interstitial changes are proportional to the degree of glomerular changes. In severe cases, cortical necrosis can be seen (12).

Secondary changes late in the course include glomerular sclerosis, either segmental or global. Reduplication of the glomerular basement membrane may occur in the late phase due to organization following endothelial injury.

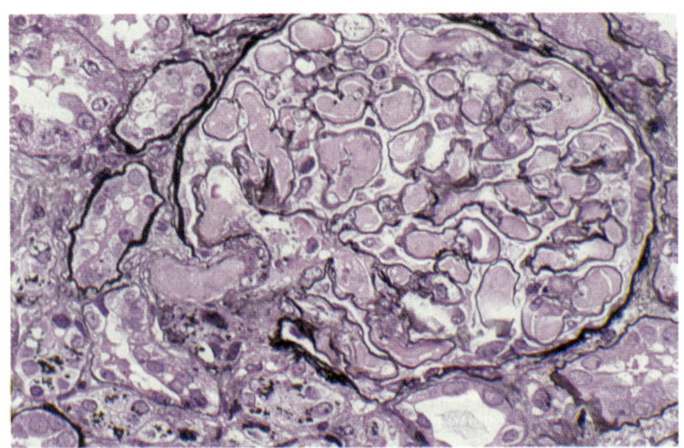

FIGURE 11.2. Entire glomerulus and arteriole are filled with chunky, eosinophilic fibrin in this case of hemolytic uremic syndrome (HUS) (Jones silver stain).

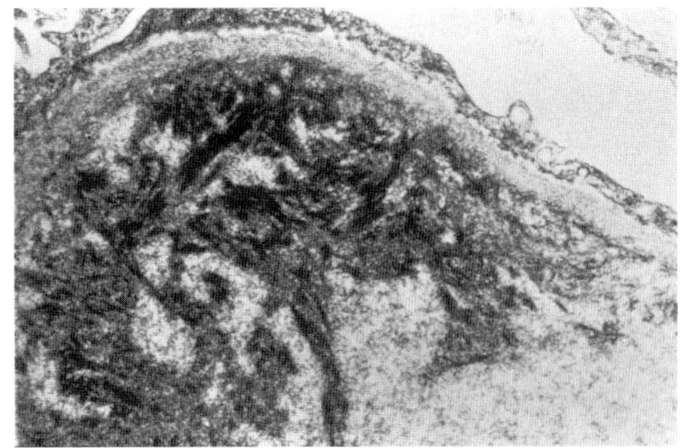

FIGURE 11.3. Fibrin tactoids in subendothelial area in thrombotic microangiopathy (electron microscopy).

Immunofluorescence Microscopy

Immunofluorescence studies show no immunoglobulin deposits. Complement and immunoglobulin M (IgM) may be present in sclerotic areas. Fibrin and fibrinogen are present in affected glomeruli and arterioles.

Electron Microscopy

Endothelial cells are frequently swollen and detachment may be seen by electron microscopy. Fibrin tactoids may be present in affected glomeruli (Fig. 11.3). Mesangiolysis is a prominent finding in early phases (11).

In the subacute and chronic phase, the increased lucency of the lamina rara interna is in part correlated to breakdown of coagulation products (Fig. 11.4). This zone contains breakdown products of fibrin, laminin, and fibronectin (2).

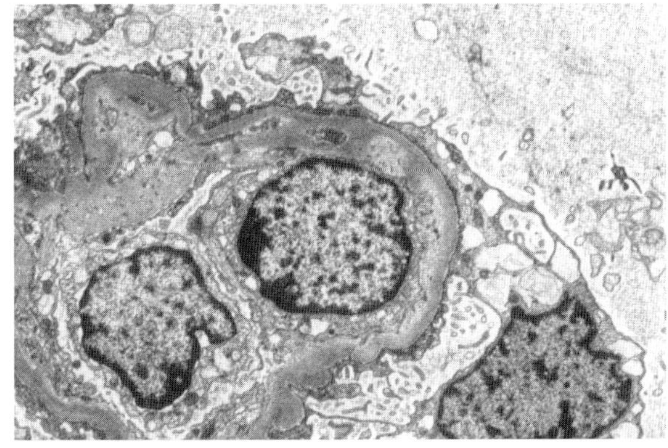

FIGURE 11.4. Increased lucency of lamina rara interna and glomerular basement membrane (GBM) corrugation in HUS (electron microscopy).

Etiology/Pathogenesis

The lesion of thrombotic microangiopathy may be seen in malignant hypertension, systemic lupus erythematosus, especially when antiphospholipid antibodies are present, pregnancy, scleroderma, and secondary to toxins and in HIV patients (8,13–16). Drugs, especially cyclosporine and mitomycin, may also cause HUS (14). Bone marrow transplant patients may develop HUS months after transplantation. In addition, genetic predisposition for thrombotic microangiopathy has been described. Familial forms of HUS and TTP occur, and are likely underrecognized (7,17,18). Familial HUS may be due to mutations in factor H, a regulator of complement, or rarely membrane cofactor protein (MCP), a cell-bound complement regulator (19). Familial TTP is due to constitutional deficiency of a von Willebrand factor–cleaving protease, whereas a nonfamilial form of TTP seems to be caused by an acquired inhibitor of this protease. This protease is now called ADAMTS13 (a member of the "*a* *d*isintegrin *a*nd *m*etalloprotease with *t*hrombo*s*pondin type 1 repeats" family of zinc metalloproteases) (7).

Common underlying infectious agents leading to hemolytic uremic syndrome have been identified. The typical diarrhea-associated (D+) form of HUS is most often associated with the shiga-like toxin or verotoxin (4,9,12). With atypical HUS (D−) no diarrheal prodrome is seen, and shiga-like toxin is not identified. Most of these infections are due to the *Escherichia coli* serotype O157:H7. Verotoxin was associated with ~90% of cases of HUS in children in North America and Europe. Undercooked hamburger meat is most closely associated with such outbreaks in North America, pointing to cattle as an important reservoir for the implicated *E. coli* serotype O157:H7. In addition, this *E. coli* strain can be transmitted from person to person, and outbreaks associated with swallowing contaminated lake water or ingestion of contaminated fruit or vegetables or cider have occurred.

The mature verotoxin has alpha and beta subunits. The beta subunits interacts with the target cell, most often the endothelial cell, binding to the glycolipid Gb3 protein. The alpha unit is cleaved and taken up by endocytosis, inactivating 60S ribosomes, thereby causing cell death. The Gb3 receptor for verotoxin is highly expressed in human kidney, perhaps underlying the susceptibility of the kidney to this toxin (19). However, Gb3 levels were not different in normal children vs. adults, so the excess risk of children for D+ HUS cannot be simply explained by overexpression of Gb3 (20).

Clinicopathologic Correlations

Histologic distribution of lesions may have some prognostic significance (see below). Age has a major impact on prognosis. Mortality of TTP in adults was nearly 100% before advent of plasma therapy. Children have a much more benign course, with less than 10% mortality even when only symptomatic treatment was given. Improved survival in the last 10 years is associated with use of a combination of antiplatelet agents and plasmapheresis (21). In some series, plasma exchange has resulted in better prognosis than plasma infusion, but the results are not clear-cut. New molecular insights (see above) suggest that plasmapheresis could be useful when acquired inhibitors of ADAMTS13 are present, whereas plasma replacement theoretically could be indicated in patients with deficiency of this protease or factor H mutation, with normal plasma presumably correcting the deficiency (19). ADAMTS13 testing has been advocated as a means to distinguish between HUS and TTP, with TTP proposed to result from ADAMTS13 mutation and resulting deficiency (7). However, there may be overlap both clinically and at a molecular level. Hemolytic uremic syndrome accounts for about half of cases of acute renal failure in HIV patients, and has a poor outcome (15). The pathogenesis of this association is not known, but animal studies do not support direct HIV infection of intrinsic renal cells as a cause of this lesion.

Long-term follow-up 10 years after HUS has shown a decrease in the glomerular filtration rate (GFR) in half of patients (22). Histologic distribution of lesions may have some prognostic significance. Degree of histologic damage, rather than initial clinical severity, was the best predictor of long-term prognosis in HUS (23). Predominantly glomerular involvement has a better outcome than larger vessel involvement. Glomerular predominant injury is the most frequent pattern of injury in children. Hypertension is more frequent with larger vessel, rather than glomerular, injury. Poor prognosis was predicted by cortical necrosis or thrombotic microangiopathy involving >50% of glomeruli at time of presentation. Segmental sclerosis was associated with decreased GFR long term. Recurrence in the transplant is very common in familial forms of HUS, and is most often associated with graft loss. Initial levels of serum plasminogen activator inhibitor-1 (PAI-1) in patients with HUS also correlated with worse long-term outcome, perhaps because high PAI-1 promotes thrombosis and also inhibits matrix breakdown (24). Recently, serum laminin P levels have been proposed to be an index of injury (25).

References

1. Symmers WSC. Thrombotic microangiopathic hemolytic anemia (thrombotic microangiopathy). Br Med J 2:897, 1952.
2. Churg J, Strauss L. Renal involvement in thrombotic microangiopathies. Semin Nephrol 5:46, 1985.
3. Goral S, Horn R, Brouillette J, Fogo A. Fever, thrombocytopenia, anasarca, and acute renal failure in a 50-year-old woman [renal biopsy teaching case]. Am J Kidney Dis 31:890–895, 1998.

4. Argyle JC, Hogg RJ, Pysher TJ, Silva FG, Siegler RL. A clinicopathological study of 24 children with hemolytic uremic syndrome. A report of the Southwest Pediatric Nephrology Study Group. Pediatr Nephrol 4:52–58, 1990.
5. Kaplan BS. The hemolytic uremic syndromes (HUS). AKF Nephrol Lett 9:29–36, 1992.
6. Kaplan BS, Cleary TG, Obrig TG. Recent advances in understanding the pathogenesis of the hemolytic uremic syndromes (Invited review). Pediatr Nephrol 4:276–283, 1990.
7. Moake JL. Thrombotic microangipathies. N Engl J Med 347:589–600, 2002.
8. Richardson SE, Karmali MA, Becker LE, Smith CR. The histopathology of the hemolytic uremic syndrome associated with verocytotoxin-producing *Escherichia coli* infections. Hum Pathol 19:1102–1108, 1988.
9. Martin DL, MacDonald KL, White KE, Soler JT, Osterholm MT. The epidemiology and clinical aspects of the hemolytic uremic syndrome in Minnesota. N Engl J Med 25:1161–1167, 1990.
10. Akashi Y, Yoshizawa N, Oshima S, et al. Hemolytic uremic syndrome without hemolytic anemia: a case report. Clin Nephrol 42:90–94, 1994.
11. Koitabashi Y, Rosenberg BF, Shapiro H, Bernstein J. Mesangiolysis: an important glomerular lesion in thrombotic microangiopathy. Mod Pathol 4:161–166, 1991.
12. Greene KD, Nichols CR, Green DP, Tauxe RV, Mottice S. Hemolytic uremic syndrome during an outbreak of *E. coli* O157:H7 infection in institutions for mentally retarded persons: clinical and epidemiological observations. J Pediatr 116:544–551, 1990.
13. Kincaid-Smith P, Nicholls K. Renal thrombotic microvascular disease associated with lupus anticoagulant. Nephron 54:285–288, 1990.
14. Zager RA. Nephrology forum: acute renal failure in the setting of bone marrow transplantation. Kidney Int 46:1443–1458, 1994.
15. Peraldi MN, Maslo C, Akposso K, Mougenot B, Rondeau E, Sraer JD. Acute renal failure in the course of HIV infection: a single-institution retrospective study of ninety-two patients anad sixty renal biopsies. Nephrol Dial Transplant 14:1578–1585, 1999.
16. Eitner F, Cui Y, Hudkins KL, et al. Thrombotic microangiopathy in the HIV-2-infected macaque. Am J Pathol 155:649–661, 1999.
17. Furlan M, Robles R, Galbusera M, et al. von Willebrand factor-cleaving protease in thrombotic thrombocytopenic purpura and the hemolytic-uremic syndrome. N Engl J Med 339:1578–1584, 1998.
18. Kaplan BS, Papadimitriou M, Brezin JH, Tomlanovich SJ, Zulkharnain. Renal transplantation in adults with autosomal recessive inheritance of hemolytic uremic syndrome. Am J Kidney Dis 30:760–765, 1997.
19. Noris M, Remuzzi G. Hemolytic uremic syndrome. J Am Soc Nephrol 16:1035–1050, 2005.
20. Ergonul Z, Clayton F, Fogo AB, Kohan DE. Shigatoxin-1 binding and receptor expression in human kidneys do not change with age. Pediatr Nephrol 18:246–253, 2003.
21. Loirat C, Sonsino E, Hinglais N, Jais JP, Landais P, Fermanian J. Treatment of the childhood hemolytic uremic syndrome with plasma. Multicenter randomized controlled clinical trial. Pediatr Nephrol 2:279–285, 1988.

22. O'Regan S, Blais N, Russo P, Pison CF, Rousseau E. Childhood hemolytic uremic syndrome: glomerular filtration rate, 6 to 11 years later, measured by 99mTc DTPA plasma slope clearance. Clin Nephrol 32:217–220, 1989.
23. Siegler RL, Milligan MK, Burningham TH, Christofferson RD, Chang SY, Jorde LB. Long-term outcome and prognostic indicators in the hemolytic-uremic syndrome. J Pediatr 118:195–200, 1991.
24. Chant ID, Milford DV, Rose PE. Plasminogen activator inhibitor activity in diarrhoea-associated haemolytic uraemic syndrome. QJM 87:737–740, 1994.
25. Segarra A, Simo R, Masmiquel L, et al. Serum concentrations of laminin-P1 in thrombotic microangiopathy: usefulness as an index of activity and prognostic value. J Am Soc Nephrol 11:434–443, 2000.

12 Diabetic Nephropathy

J. CHARLES JENNETTE

Introduction/Clinical Setting

Diabetic nephropathy is a clinical syndrome in a patient with diabetes mellitus that is characterized by persistent albuminuria, worsening proteinuria, hypertension, and progressive renal failure (1,2). Approximately a third of patients with type 1 insulin-dependent diabetes mellitus (IDDM) and type 2 non–insulin-dependent diabetes mellitus (NIDDM) develop diabetic nephropathy (2). The pathologic hallmark of diabetic nephropathy is diabetic glomerulosclerosis that results from a progressive increase in extracellular matrix in the glomerular mesangium and glomerular basement membranes. Diabetic glomerulosclerosis is the leading cause of end-stage renal disease in the United States, Europe, and Japan (1).

Pathologic Findings

Light Microscopy

Diabetic nephropathy causes pathologic abnormalities in all of the major structural compartments of the kidney, including the glomeruli, extraglomerular vessels, interstitium, and tubules (3–10).

The earliest glomerular change is enlargement (hypertrophy, hyperplasia, glomerulomegaly), which corresponds to the early clinical phase of elevated glomerular filtration rate. By the time albuminuria is detectable, there is generalized thickening of glomerular basement membranes (GBMs) and an increase in mesangial matrix material. In the earliest phase, morphometry is required to detect these changes, but eventually the GBM thickening and mesangial expansion is so pronounced that it can be readily discerned by routine light microscopy, especially if a special stain that accentuates collagenous structures is used [e.g., periodic acid-schiff (PAS), Jones silver, Masson trichrome]. Mild mesangial hypercellularity occasionally accompanies the matrix expansion; thus, care must be taken

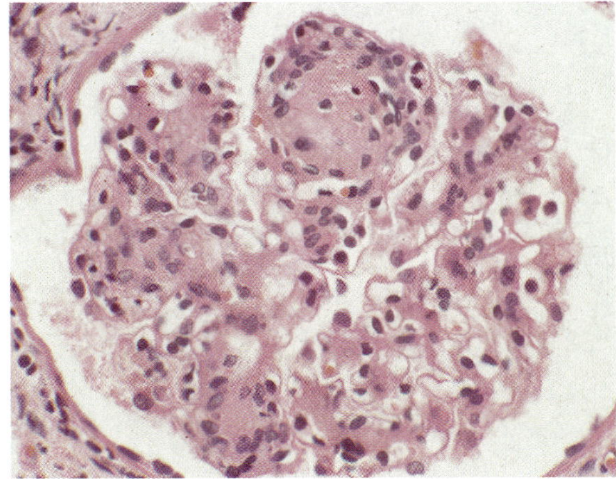

FIGURE 12.1. Glomerulus from patient with diabetic glomerulosclerosis showing segmental mesangial matrix expansion and hypercellularity that is most pronounced on the left. The upper pole has a Kimmelstiel-Wilson (K-W) nodule [hematoxylin and eosin (H&E) stain].

not to misdiagnose early diabetic glomerulosclerosis as mesangioproliferative glomerulonephritis.

Overt glomerular mesangial matrix expansion (glomerulosclerosis) manifests as diffuse mesangial matrix expansion or nodular mesangial matrix expansion or, most often, a combination of both (Figs. 12.1 to 12.5).

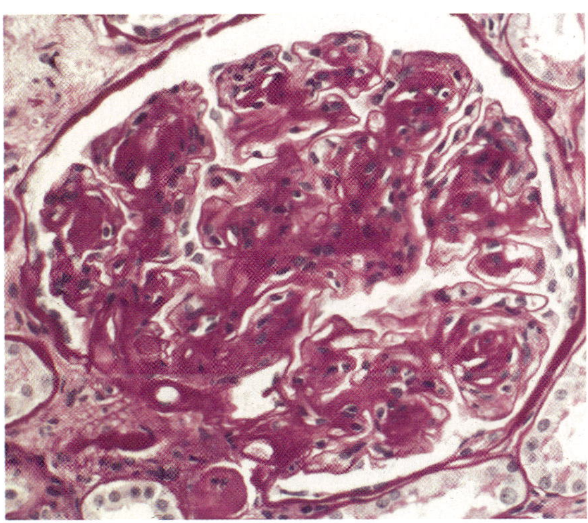

FIGURE 12.2. Glomerulus from patient with diabetic glomerulosclerosis showing relatively diffuse mesangial matrix expansion, although there is slight nodularity in some segments [periodic acid-schiff (PAS) stain].

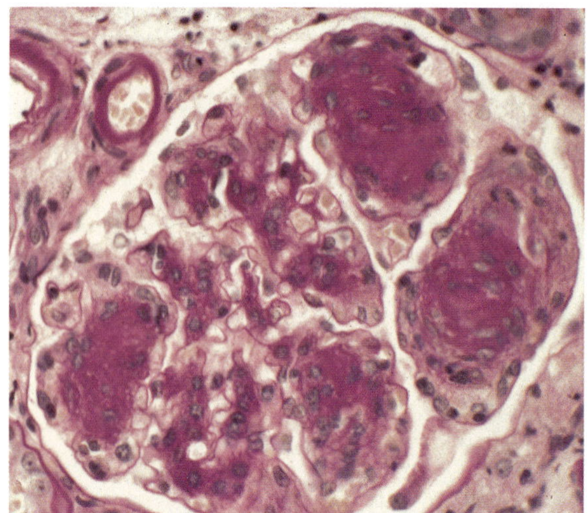

FIGURE 12.3. Glomerulus from patient with diabetic glomerulosclerosis showing multiple K-W nodules (PAS stain). The afferent and efferent arterioles in the upper left corner both have PAS-positive hyalinosis.

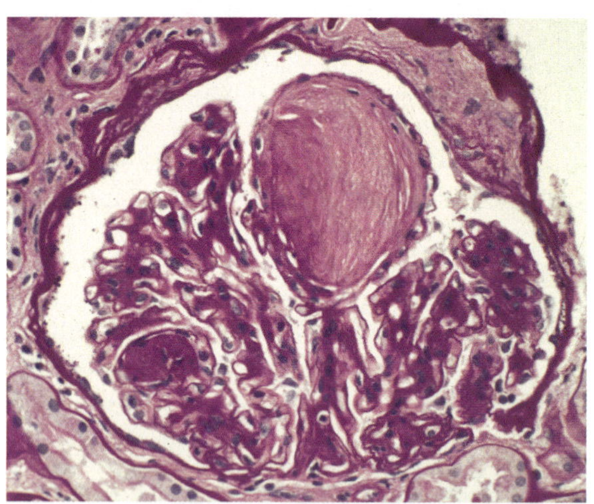

FIGURE 12.4. Glomerulus from patient with diabetic glomerulosclerosis showing a large K-W nodule with vague lamination (PAS stain).

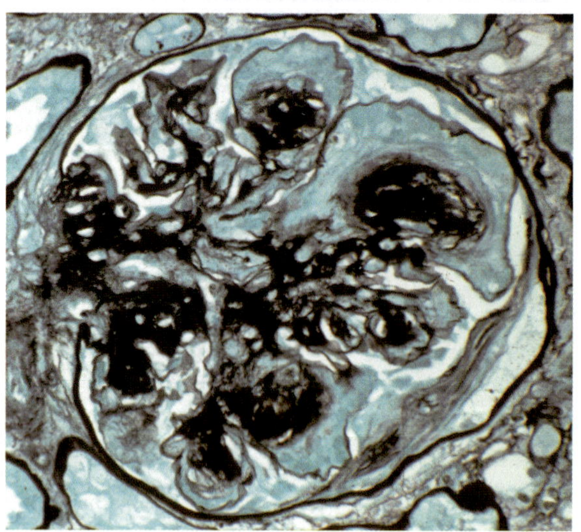

FIGURE 12.5. Glomerulus from patient with diabetic glomerulosclerosis showing extensive capillary aneurysm formation as a result of mesangiolysis that has released the GBM from the mesangium (Jones silver stain).

Glomerular basement membrane thickening usually accompanies the mesangial matrix expansion, but it may be somewhat discordant in severity (4). The designations *diffuse* versus *nodular glomerulosclerosis* are primarily of descriptive value in the biopsy report and have no value in the diagnosis because the distinctions do not have clinical significance.

Diffuse diabetic glomerulosclerosis is less specific for diabetic glomerulosclerosis than nodular diabetic glomerulosclerosis. Especially if the clinical presence of diabetes is not known and there is accompanying mesangial hypercellularity, the light microscopic changes can be mistaken for a mesangioproliferative glomerulonephritis. Careful examination may reveal early mesangial nodules, which will suggest the correct diagnosis.

The nodular lesions of diabetic glomerulosclerosis were first described by Kimmelstiel and Wilson (3) and thus are called Kimmelstiel-Wilson (K-W) nodules. The nodules begin in the heart of the mesangial region of a segment. As the nodule of matrix accrues, there may be increased numbers of mesangial cells, especially at its leading edges (Fig. 12.1). The nodules often are focal and segmental, although occasional specimens have rather diffuse global nodularity. The nodules have the same tinctorial properties as normal mesangial matrix, and thus are PAS and silver positive (Figs. 12.3 to 12.5). The matrix at the center of the nodules may be homogeneous or laminated (Fig. 12.4). K-W nodules may have a corona of capillary aneurysms that are formed as a result of mesangiolysis, which disrupts the attachment points of the GBM to the mesangium (Fig. 12.5).

Glomerular hyalinosis is common in diabetic glomerulosclerosis. These hyaline lesions may result from insudation or exudation of plasma proteins from vessels followed by entrapment in matrix. The hyalinosis can occur anywhere in the tuft, but there are two characteristic patterns: hyaline caps and capsular drops. The hyaline caps are produced when the hyalinosis forms arcs at the periphery of segments, sometimes appearing to fill the capillary aneurysms. Capsular drops are spherical accumulations of hyaline material adjacent to or within Bowman's capsule.

Crescent formation is identified in <5% of specimens with diabetic glomerulosclerosis (Fig. 12.6). When crescents are observed, one should consider the possibility of a concurrent glomerulonephritis that is more often associated with crescents, such as antineutrophil cytoplasmic antibodies (ANCA) disease or anti-GBM disease.

Diabetic glomerulosclerosis is caused by both type 1 (IDDM) and type 2 (NIDDM). The latter is somewhat more heterogeneous in appearance (5,8), in part because it often is altered by concurrent hypertensive and aging changes. At a comparable stage of diabetic nephropathy, the glomerular lesions in type 2 diabetes tend to be less severe than those in type 1 (7).

Arteriolosclerosis and arteriosclerosis are typical accompaniments to diabetic glomerulosclerosis. Arteriolar hyalinosis at the glomerular hilum

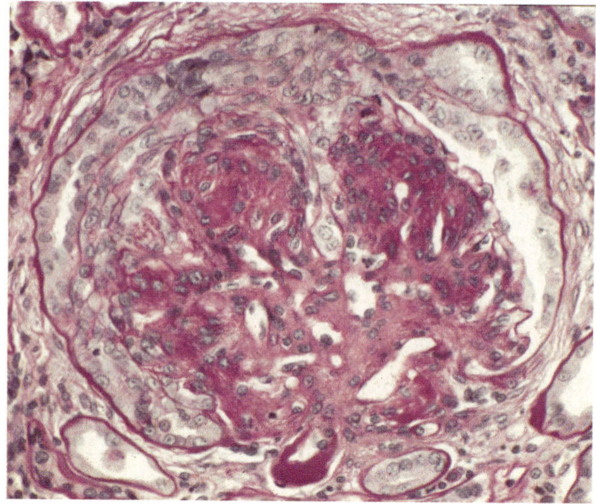

FIGURE 12.6. Glomerulus from patient with diabetic glomerulosclerosis showing cellular crescent formation (PAS stain). No other glomerular disease was identified. Note the hyalinosis of the efferent arteriole.

is ubiquitous with diabetic glomerulosclerosis and typically affects both the afferent and efferent arterioles (10). Hypertensive hyaline arteriolar sclerosis affects the afferent but not efferent arteriole.

The earliest tubular change is thickening of tubular basement membranes (TBMs) that is analogous to the GBM thickening (Fig. 12.7). With

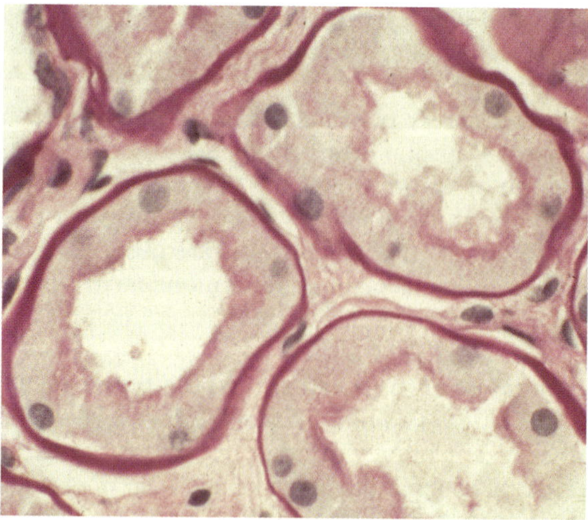

FIGURE 12.7. Proximal tubules from patient with diabetic glomerulosclerosis showing markedly thickened tubular basement membranes even though there is no tubular atrophy or interstitial fibrosis (PAS stain).

progressive chronic disease, tubules become atrophic and the interstitium develops fibrosis and chronic inflammation. Except for the marked TBM thickening, these chronic tubulointerstitial changes resemble those seen with any form of progressive glomerular disease.

Immunofluorescence Microscopy

Typical diabetic glomerulosclerosis usually can be diagnosed with reasonable accuracy from the immunofluorescence microscopy findings alone. The characteristic feature is linear staining of GBMs with antisera specific for immunoglobulin G (IgG) and other plasma proteins, although the staining for IgG is usually brightest (Fig. 12.8). Kappa light chain staining usually is brighter than lambda light chain staining. Immunofluorescence microscopy is useful for ruling out other glomerular diseases that can mimic diabetic glomerulosclerosis by light microscopy, such as monoclonal immunoglobulin deposition disease, membranoproliferative glomerulonephritis, fibrillary glomerulonephritis, and amyloidosis. Bowman's capsule and TBMs also often show linear staining.

In addition to the linear staining for IgG, the background fluorescence often allows identification of the typical nodular sclerosis because the mesangial nodules may also stain for IgG and other determinants.

The overall histology, not to mention the clinical features, usually preclude any confusion with anti-GBM disease as a result of the linear GBM staining for IgG.

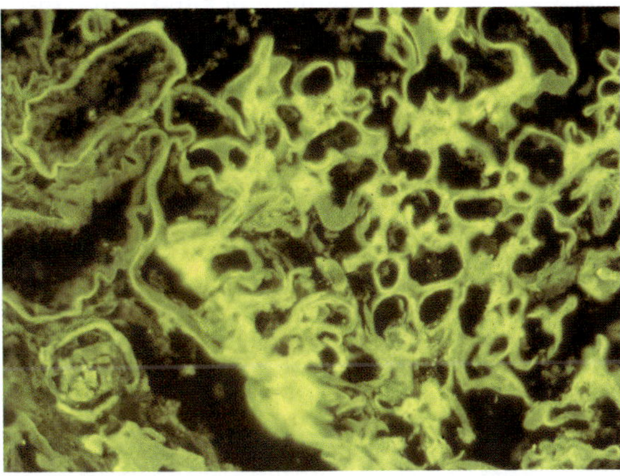

FIGURE 12.8. Glomerulus from patient with diabetic glomerulosclerosis showing linear staining of glomerular basement membranes (GBMs) by immunofluorescence microscopy for immunoglobulin G (IgG). Note also the tubular basement membrane (TBM) staining on the left.

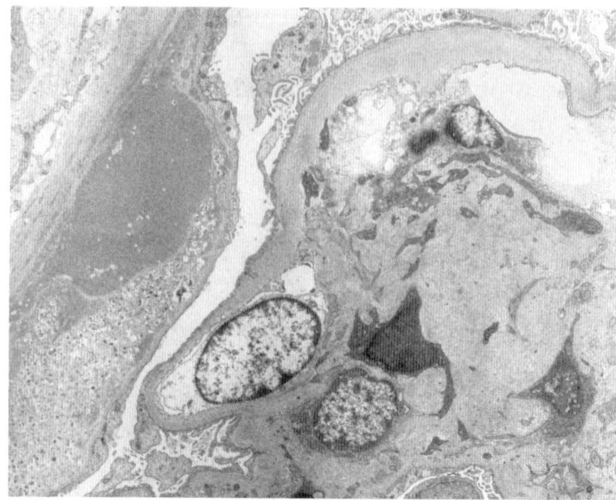

FIGURE 12.9. Electron microscopy of a glomerulus from patient with diabetic glomerulosclerosis showing marked increase in mesangial matrix (lower right quadrant), thickening of the GBM (especially at the top of the image), and a capsular drop of electron-dense insudative material (upper left quadrant).

Electron Microscopy

Ultrastructural examination confirms the structural abnormalities seen by light microscopy (4,9) and helps document that there is no other glomerular disease that is mimicking diabetic glomerulosclerosis by light microscopy. For example, monoclonal immunoglobulin deposition disease would have granular densities in the GBM, membranoproliferative glomerulonephritis would have subendothelial or intramembranous dense deposits, and fibrillary glomerulonephritis or amyloidosis would have deposits with a distinctive fibrillary substructure.

The typical finding is thickening of GBMs and mesangial matrix expansion (Fig. 12.9) (9). The protein insudation (hyalinosis by light microscopy) appears as electron-dense material and should not be misinterpreted as immune complex deposits. In line with the distribution of hyaline seen by light microscopy, this electron dense insudative material may occur as capsular drops in Bowman's capsule (Fig. 12.9) or as extensive dense accumulations in aneurysmal capillaries forming caps on mesangial nodules. Arterioles with hyalinosis by light microscopy have extensive deposition of insudative homogeneous electron-dense material by electron microscopy (9,10).

Etiology/Pathogenesis

The etiology and pathogenesis of diabetic nephropathy is multifactorial (2,11,12). Contributing factors could influence both the susceptibility to and the rate of progression of diabetic nephropathy include genetic, metabolic, hemodynamic, and structural characteristics. Although the etiology of the diabetes is very different in type 1 and type 2 diabetes mellitus, the basic pathophysiologic events that lead to the nephropathy probably are very similar in both (12).

The importance of genetic factors is indicated by the observation that only about a third of diabetic patients develop nephropathy and that this is independent of the severity or control of hyperglycemia (2). Some but not all of the genes that have been implicated in affecting the susceptibility for or progression of diabetic nephropathy are promoter of RAGE (advanced glycation end-product receptor), histocompatibility antigen DR3/4, angiotensin-converting enzyme, angiotensinogen, bradykinin receptor, aldose reductase, transforming growth factor-β, and apolipoprotein E (12).

Experimental data indicate that many different cell types in all structural compartments of the kidney are stimulated by hyperglycemia and other stimuli (e.g., advanced glycation end products and reactive oxygen species) to produce cytokines, growth factors (e.g., transforming growth factor-β, platelet-derived growth factor-β) and other humoral mediators that cause increased extracellular matrix production (2,11,12). Activation of the renin-angiotensin system by high glucose and altered hemodynamics (e.g., reduced blood flow caused by narrowed arteries, arterioles, and capillaries) also contribute to many pathophysiologic events including increased extracellular matrix accumulation (11,12).

Monoclonal immunoglobulin deposition disease (MIDD) may provide insight into the pathogenesis of diabetic glomerulosclerosis. It is caused by the deposition of monoclonal immunoglobulin light chains or heavy chains or both in GBMs and mesangial matrix, resulting in nodular glomerulosclerosis that is identical to diabetic glomerulosclerosis by light microscopy. This suggests that the IgG localization in GBMs in diabetic glomerulosclerosis may be the cause of the nodular sclerosis and not merely an epiphenomenon.

Clinicopathologic Correlations

Clinical manifestations of diabetic nephropathy do not occur until overt structural features of diabetic glomerulosclerosis have developed (4).

Patients with type 1 or type 2 diabetic nephropathy have a variable rate of decline in glomerular filtration rate that usually falls between 1 to 2 mL/min/year (median 12 mL/min/year) (1). Proteinuria increases progressively, with approximately 50% of patients becoming nephrotic. There is a strong correlation between the severity of diabetic glomerulosclerosis and the severity and progression of renal insufficiency and proteinuria (4,6). One hypothesis for the correlation between glomerular sclerosis and reduced renal function is that the mesangial expansion impinges on the capillary lumen and reduces the filtering surface area, which in turn reduces the glomerular filtration rate (4,11). The severity of arteriolar hyalinosis also parallels the severity of glomerulosclerosis and has a positive correlation with severity of proteinuria and renal insufficiency (10). Severity of proteinuria correlates better with mesangial matrix expansion than with GBM thickening (4). Proteinuria in diabetic nephropathy may result more from direct toxic effects on podocytes than from alterations in the GBM alone (11).

Diabetic glomerulosclerosis recurs in renal allografts from 2 to 10 years after transplantation (13,14). In patients with type 1 diabetes, simultaneous pancreatic transplantation can protect against recurrent diabetic nephropathy. The earliest and most frequent change is arteriolar hyalinosis. Linear GBM staining for IgG also is an early marker of recurrence. Less than 10% of kidneys develop overt nodular sclerosis.

Because hypertension, dyslipidemia, and poor glycemic control are important risk factors for progression of diabetic nephropathy, combined therapies to control these factors (including angiotensin-converting enzyme inhibitors or angiotensin receptor blockers) is the current management strategy for diabetic nephropathy (15). In patients with type 1 diabetes mellitus, pancreas transplantation can reverse the pathologic lesions of diabetic nephropathy, although reversal requires more than 5 years of normoglycemia (16).

References

1. Parving HH. Diabetic nephropathy: prevention and treatment. Kidney Int 60:2041–2055, 2001.
2. Schena FP, Gesualdo L. Pathogenetic mechanisms of diabetic nephropathy. J Am Soc Nephrol 16:S30–S33, 2005.
3. Kimmelstiel P, Wilson C. Intercapillary lesions in glomeruli of kidney. Am J Pathol 12:83–97, 1936.
4. Mauer SM, Staffes MV, Ellis EN, Sutherland DE, Brown DM, Goetz FC. Structural-functional relationships in diabetic nephropathy. J Clin Invest 74:1143–1154, 1984.
5. Gambara V, Mecca G, Remuzzi G, Bertani T. Heterogeneous nature of renal lesions in type II diabetes. J Am Soc Nephrol 3:1458–1466, 1993.
6. Østerby R, Gall MA, Schmitz A, Nielsen FS, Nyberg G, Parving HH. Glomerular structure and function in proteinuric type-2 (non-insulin-dependent) diabetic patients. Diabetologia 36:1064–1070, 1993.
7. Bertani T, Gambara V, Remuzzi G. Structural basis of diabetic nephropathy in microalbuminuric NIDDM patients: a light microscopy study. Diabetologia 39:1625–1628, 1996.
8. Fioretto P, Mauer M, Brocco E, et al. Patterns of renal injury in NIDDM patients with microalbuminuria. Diabetologia 39:1569–1576, 1996.
9. Østerby R. Renal changes in the diabetic kidney. Nephrol Dial Transplant 12:1282–1283, 1997.
10. Østerby R, Hartmann A, Bangstad HJ. Structural changes in renal arterioles in type 1 diabetic patients. Diabetología 45:542–549, 2002.

11. Adler S. Diabetic nephropathy: linking histology, cell biology, and genetics. Kidney Int 66:2095–2106, 2004.
12. Wolf G. New insights into the pathophysiology of diabetic nephropathy: from haemodynamics to molecular pathology. Eur J Clin Invest 34:785–796, 2004.
13. Bohman SO, Wilczek H, Tyden G, Jaremko G, Lundgren G, Groth CG. Recurrent diabetic nephropathy in renal allografts placed in diabetic patients and protective effect of simultaneous pancreatic transplantation. Transplant Proc 19:2290–2293, 1987.
14. Salifu MO, Nicastri AD, Markell MS, Ghali H, Sommer BG, Friedman EA. Allograft diabetic nephropathy may progress to end-stage renal disease. Pediatr Transplant 8:351–356, 2004.
15. Fioretto P, Solini A. Antihypertensive treatment and multifactorial approach for renal protection in diabetes. J Am Soc Nephrol 16:S18–21, 2005.
16. Fioretto P, Steffes MW, Sutherland DE, Goetz FC, Mauer M. Reversal of lesions of diabetic nephropathy after pancreas transplantation. N Engl J Med 339:69–75, 1998.

Section VI
Tubulointerstitial Diseases

13
Acute Interstitial Nephritis

Arthur H. Cohen

Introduction/Clinical Setting

Acute interstitial nephritis (AIN) may be the result of indirect injury by drugs, reaction to systemic infections, direct renal infection (viral and selected bacteria), humoral immune responses (anti–tubular basement membrane disease), hereditary and metabolic disorders, and obstruction and reflux in the acute stages. Similar changes can also be observed in the kidney in systemic diseases such as lupus erythematosus and in transplant rejection. Acute tubulointerstitial nephritis also occurs to varying degrees in association with glomerulonephritides. This section is largely confined to the drug-induced, reactive, idiopathic and immunologic disorders inducing AIN. Acute interstitial nephritis usually presents with acute renal failure, often oliguric; it is sometimes associated with systemic manifestations such as arthralgia fever, eosinophilia and rash, typically as a consequence of drug hypersensitivity (1–3).

Pathologic Findings

On gross examination, kidneys with AIN are enlarged with a pale cortex and a distinct corticomedullary junction. Histologically there is diffuse interstitial edema with an interstitial infiltrate of lymphocytes, monocyte-macrophages, and plasma cells to varying degrees (Fig. 13.1). Eosinophils may comprise from 0% to 10% of the infiltrate, depending on the etiology of the AIN. When there are many eosinophils, they may be focally concentrated. The inflammatory cells are often prominent at the corticomedullary junction, and are generally confined to the cortex. Neutrophils and basophils are infrequent; large numbers of neutrophils suggest a diagnosis of acute infectious interstitial nephritis. In some cases granulomas may be found in the interstitium or around ruptured tubules. Glomeruli and vessels are usually uninvolved. The inflammation extends into the walls and lumina of tubules (tubulitis), with distal tubules more often affected than

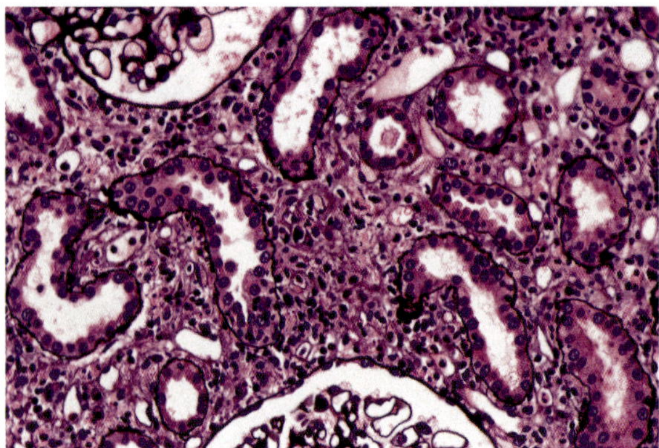

Figure 13.1. The interstitium is edematous (tubules with normal basement membranes are separated) and infiltrated by lymphocytes, some of which are in the walls of tubules [periodic acid-schiff (PAS) stain].

proximal tubules. There are varying numbers of degenerating and regenerating tubular epithelial cells; occasionally desquamated cells may be observed in tubular lumina. Proximal tubules often have focal loss of brush border staining. Immunofluorescent studies are usually negative but infrequently reveal granular deposits of complement in the tubular basement membranes (TBMs) and rarely fibrin in the interstitium. In cases of anti-TBM antibody formation, there is linear staining of TBMs for immunoglobulin G (IgG).

Etiology/Pathogenesis

Acute interstital nephritis is a morphologic entity with many pathogenetic etiologies. These include cell-mediated immunity of the delayed hypersensitivity type and possibly direct cytotoxicity, humoral immunity such as anti-TBM antibody formation, and others possibly including complement activation and enhanced expression of major histocompatibility complex (MHC) class I or class II antigens. Some studies have reported drug-induced acute interstitial nephritis to represent approximately 6.5% of nontransplant biopsies. Delayed hypersensitivity is the likely mechanism for AIN induced by drugs, particularly antibiotics and nonsteroidal antiinflammatory drugs (NSAIDs). T cells carrying both CD4 and CD8 antigens in varying proportions have been identified in kidneys with drug-induced AIN. This variability may be related to the offending agent or the time course of the biopsy. The T cells have been shown to carry activation markers and therefore are presumed to be effector cells in the hypersensitivity process. B cells are also present to some extent, more so with NSAID-induced AIN. This allergic form of AIN may be associated with a granulomatous response, particularly with sulfa-containing drugs and oxacillin, although it has been reported with a number of medications. Delayed hypersensitivity is currently the most favored mechanism for the majority of drug-induced episodes of AIN, and may be related to fixed antigens (drugs, metabolites, or either of these bound to tissue components, or altered tissue components). This response is idiosyncratic and is not dose-related, although it may require up to 1 year of use to occur with NSAIDs. Other actions of drugs such as the nonsteroidals that result in acute renal failure include direct toxicity or functional abnormalities related to alterations in prostaglandin synthesis. Hypersensitivity may also account for the occurrence of AIN in kidneys of patients with systemic streptococcal, diphtheria, or measles infections in the absence of direct renal infection. This is more of historical importance as its occurrence is infrequent now; it produces a picture similar to that of the more often occurring drug-associated AIN.

Humoral immunity is a less frequent but in some ways better understood mechanism resulting in AIN. Rodent models of anti-TBM disease have been characterized by linear staining of TBMs with IgG and C3 with associated interstitial mononuclear inflammation, giant cells and edema, and tubular damage. The humoral immune role has been shown by the passive transfer of this process in animals with immune serum but not with immune cells.

In the setting of AIN, anti-TBM antibody formation is most often a secondary process and likely not responsible for significant renal injury. These antibodies are probably produced when drugs interact with a portion of the TBM, which macrophages then digest, presenting a new autoantigen; several antigens ranging from 48 to 70 kd are potential targets of the anti-TBM antibodies. Anti-TBM disease is rare. Anti-TBM antibodies uncommonly occur in association with membranous glomerulonephritis and may be genetically determined. Reaginic antibodies uncommonly may be induced during infections or by other agents and cross-react with renal elements, or form immune complexes that deposit in the renal tubules or interstitium. Other suggested mechanisms for the induction of AIN include enhanced expression of MHC antigens on renal cells such as tubular epithelium. Interferon and other cytokines associated with immunologically mediated processes are known to upregulate MHC expression, possibly eliciting an inflammatory response. Complement activation has been proposed as a possible source of continuing injury in AIN. Granular immune complex deposits in TBMs are common in systemic lupus erythematosus and when present invariably are accompanied by lupus immune complex glomerulonephritis. On the other hand, isolated TBM deposits are a feature of Sjögren's syndrome. Recently, another group of patients with extensive tubulointerstitial deposits with associated hypocomplementemia was described; it was suggested that this resulted from local immune complex formation.

Microscopic features reported as portending a worse prognosis in acute interstitial nephritis include presence of tubular atrophy with interstitial fibrosis, interstitial granulomata, and a greater inflammatory infiltrate.

Clinicopathologic Correlations

Acute renal failure is correlated with interstitial edema and inflammation as well as tubular inflammation with associated acute tubular cell injury up to 60% of patients require dialysis (4). Proteinuria is usually modest in the range of 1.0 g/24 hours except when combined with minimal change disease as a consequence of NSAIDs or other drug-induced damage. In these instances nephrotic range proteinuria is observed (5). The renal outcome, with or without corticosteroid therapy, is generally good. Modest stable chronic renal insufficiency is common, reflecting resolution of the acute inflammatory process (4).

References

1. Rastegar A, Kashgarian M. The clinical-spectrum of tubulo-interstitial nephritis. Kidney Int 54:313–327, 1998.
2. Michel DM, Kelly CJ. Acute interstitial nephritis. J Am Soc Nephrol 9:506–515, 1998.
3. Cavallo T. Tubulo-interstitial nephritis. In: Jennette JC, Olson JL, Schwartz MM, Silva FG, eds. Heptinstall's Pathology of the Kidney, 5th ed. Philadelphia: Lippincott-Raven, 1998:667–724.
4. Clarkson MR, Giblin L, O'Connell FP, et al. Acute interstitial nephritis: clinical features and response to corticosteroid therapy. Nephrol Dial Transplant 19:2778–2783, 2004.
5. Markowitz GS, Perazella MA. Drug-induced renal failure: a focus on tubulointerstitial disease. Clin Chim Acta 351:31–47, 2005.

14
Chronic Interstitial Nephritis

Arthur H. Cohen

Introduction/Clinical Setting

Chronic interstitial nephritis represents a large and diverse group of disorders characterized primarily by interstitial fibrosis with mononuclear leukocyte infiltration and tubular atrophy (1–3). The chronic damage is unrelated to underlying glomerular or vascular processes. Among the many causes of chronic interstitial nephritis are high-grade vesicoureteral reflux, urinary obstruction, chronic bacterial infections, Sjögren's syndrome, drugs (lithium, Chinese herbs), radiation, and Balkan nephropathy (3). Although the pathologic aspects by light microscopy have the above-mentioned features in common, historical information, imaging data, familial history, and gross pathology features may help to distinguish one disease from another. Because it was once widely considered that most chronic interstitial nephritis represented chronic infection, the term *chronic pyelonephritis* was commonly used for this group of disorders (1,2). However, chronic pyelonephritis is a rare entity (4).

Pathologic Findings

Gross Findings

As high-grade reflux is such an important and representative form of chronic interstitial nephritis, it alone will be the focus of this discussion. When examined grossly, the kidney in patients with reflux and chronic interstitial nephritis (also called reflux nephropathy) has scarring primarily at the poles with dilated calyces and overlying thinned pale parenchyma. These areas have irregular, broad, deep scars with contraction. The other areas of kidney may not be affected, or may have a finely granular surface indicating ischemic effect. The walls of the affected calyces and pelvis are thickened. In contrast, with obstruction there are diffuse pelvicalyceal dilatation and uniform parenchymal thinning. Calculi may or may not be

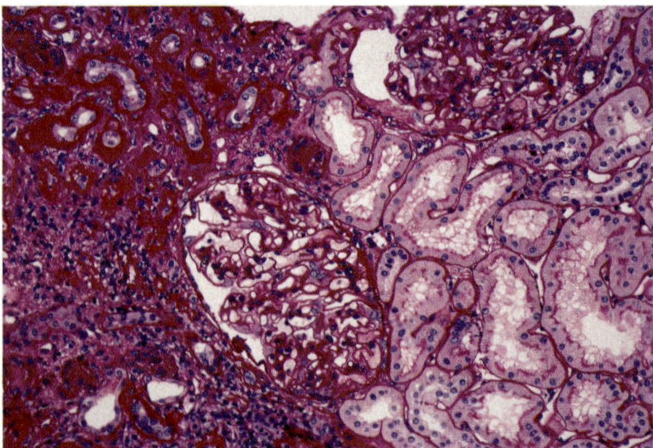

FIGURE 14.1. In this low-magnification photograph, there is a large area of tubular atrophy, interstitial fibrosis, and lymphocytic infiltration; few completely sclerotic glomeruli are present [periodic acid-schiff (PAS) stain].

evident. The renal surface is smooth or finely granular with only shallow scars induced by ischemia.

Light Microscopy

Microscopically, there is tubular atrophy with associated interstitial fibrosis, with areas of tubular dropout in more severe cases. Foci of thinned dilated tubules containing cast material may be seen (thyroidization), particularly in the outer cortex. Tubules focally are ruptured, and Tamm-Horsfall protein with other intraluminal contents is in extratubular locations. Mononuclear inflammatory cells including lymphocytes, histiocytes, and plasma cells are throughout the interstitium in large numbers (Figs. 14.1 and 14.2); lymphoid follicles may be observed. If active infection

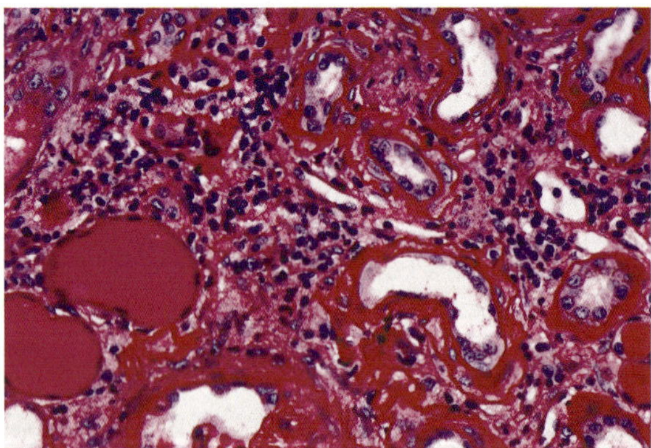

FIGURE 14.2. Lymphocytes are in the fibrotic interstitium and in walls of some atrophied tubules (PAS stain).

is still present, neutrophils and a small number of eosinophils may also be found. The calyces and pelvis disclose mononuclear leukocytes, fibrosis, and hypertrophy of the smooth muscle; the overlying transitional epithelium may be hyperplastic or display glandular or squamous metaplasia. Renal arteries often have intimal fibrosis and muscular hypertrophy, while glomeruli show ischemic collapse and periglomerular fibrosis. Glomeruli may have Tamm-Horsfall protein in Bowman's space. In severe reflux nephropathy, there is hypertrophy of the glomeruli and tubules in the nonscarred parenchyma; there is sharp demarcation between the scarred and preserved parenchyma. Enlarged glomeruli may also demonstrate focal and segmental glomerulosclerosis. Some investigators have reported that in nonscarred areas, glomeruli with elongated capillaries, adhesions, and podocyte detachment were associated with a poorer prognosis (5).

Etiology/Pathogenesis

Reflux nephropathy has been extensively studied in a pig experimental model; the pig has been used because it has compound papillae at the renal poles as humans do. Radiographic and pathologic studies have demonstrated that refluxing urine can gain access to the parenchyma in these locations. The compound papillae have large ducts of Bellini into which refluxed material can enter; the broad openings of these ducts do not prevent this process as the smaller more angulated duct openings of simple papillae do. The refluxing urine can induce tubular rupture with extravasation of the tubular contents, or may cause forniceal tears with direct extension of urine into the parenchyma. This process of pyelotubular backflow is known as intrarenal reflux. There is local damage in response to the extravasated material, with scar formation occurring within 1 to 2 weeks in the pig model. While some investigators have proposed that the urinary contents alone are adequate to induce scar formation, it is more widely believed that some element of infection is required to produce chronic interstitial nephritis. Refluxing urine, usually resulting from inadequate length or abnormal positioning of the ureterovesical junction orifice, is a common mechanism. Studies suggest that nitric oxide stimulated by macrophage colony-stimulating factor may be a major mediator of tissue damage in reflux nephropathy (6). Children under the age of 5 have shorter ureters and more patent ducts of Bellini, and therefore are more prone to develop reflux nephropathy. In fact, many polar scars occur prior to the age of 4 or 5 years, and do not substantially worsen after that time as the intravesical ureter lengthens and reflux subsides. As the scarring occurs, a component of arterial intimal fibrosis often ensues, with additional damage resulting from ischemia.

References

1. Risdon RA. Pyelonephritis and feflux nephropathy. In: Tischer CC, Brenner BM, eds. Renal Pathology with Clinical and Functional Correlations, 2nd ed. Philadelphia: Lippincott, 1994: 832–862.
2. Heptinstall RH. Urinary tract infection, pyelonephritis, reflux nephropathy. In: Jennette JC, Olson JL, Schwartz MM, Silva FG, eds. Heptinstall's Pathology of the Kidney, 5th ed. Philadelphia: Lippincott-Raven, 1998:725–784.
3. van Ypersele de Strihou C, Vanderweghen JL. The tragic paradigm of Chinese herbs nephropathy. Nephrol Dial Transplant 10:157–160, 1995.
4. Hill GS. Calcium and the kidney, hydronephrosis. In: Jennette JC, Olson JL, Schwartz MM, Silva FG, eds. Heptinstall's Pathology of the Kidney, 5th ed. Philadelphia: Lippincott-Raven, 1998:891–936.
5. Rolle U, Shima H, Puri P. Nitric oxide, enhanced by macrophage-colony stimulating factor, mediates renal damage in reflux nephropathy. Kidney Int 62:507–513, 2002.
6. Tada M, Jimi S, Hisano S, et al. Histopathological evidence of poor prognosis in patients with vesicoureteral reflux. Pediatr Nephrol 16:482–487, 2001.

15 Acute Tubular Necrosis

Arthur H. Cohen

Introduction/Clinical Setting

Acute tubular necrosis (ATN) is a pathologic process that manifests clinically as acute renal failure. Although the term implies cellular death (necrosis), it should be appreciated that frank necrosis is not a constant finding; evidence of sublethal cellular injury is common. Furthermore, there is often a lack of clinical-pathologic correlation, with severe acute renal failure sometimes associated with trivial morphologic findings (1,2).

Broadly speaking, ATN may be the result of one of two mechanisms: ischemia or toxin induced. The structural changes in each are reasonably distinctive, and pathogenic mechanisms are also considered different. Traditionally, ischemic ATN follows hypotension or hypovolemia or both (3,4). There may be many causes of this circulatory state; these include extensive trauma with rhabdomyolysis and myoglobinuria, incompatible blood transfusions, pancreatitis, septic shock in a variety of settings, extensive hemolysis as in malaria (blackwater fever), and shock following administration of barbiturates, morphine, and sedatives. Toxic ATN is a dose-dependent injury with extensive tubular cell necrosis normally limited to a specific portion of the nephron and usually involving almost all nephrons. This is obviously in sharp contrast to ischemic tubular necrosis in which the changes are considerably more subtle and patchy. Many therapeutic and diagnostic agents, industrial chemicals, heavy metals, and plants may be responsible for this lesion. The classic agent is mercuric chloride; the changes are quite prominent and impressive.

Ischemic Acute Tubular Necrosis

Light Microscopy

The pathologic changes in ischemic ATN are often subtle but are easily discernible with well-fixed tissue. Both proximal and distal tubules are affected. The proximal tubules are dilated and the lining cells flattened.

Brush border staining is reduced or absent (Fig. 15.1). This combination of changes causes proximal tubules to resemble distal tubules ("distalization") and is also known as simplification of tubules so that one nephron segment cannot easily be differentiated from another. Distal tubules, including the thick ascending limb of Henle, are dilated and lined by flattened cells. Tamm-Horsfall protein containing casts, sometimes incorporating granular material, are frequently present but are not specific for ATN. In addition, pigmented (tan-brown) granular casts are characteristic; many studies have concluded that heme pigment is responsible for this appearance. Oxalate crystals are commonly present and are located in the thick ascending limb, distal tubule, and collecting duct. It should be noted that the crystals are usually not numerous; marked accumulation of oxalate crystals is most commonly observed in ethylene glycol poisoning. Overt or extensive necrosis of tubular cells is neither common nor regularly observed. Instead, loss of individual cells, manifested by incomplete epithelial lining of tubules, is present. This change requires well-fixed tissue and a practiced eye to demonstrate. It is often referred to as the "nonreplacement" phenomenon. There are often desquamated cells or cellular debris in the lumina (Fig. 15.2).

Ischemic tubular necrosis is frequently associated with disruption of tubular walls (including cell loss and basement membrane disruption) with spillage of contents into the adjacent interstitium. It also may be associated with localized inflammation, sometimes in the form of granulomata. However, inflammation is not constantly present. The interstitium is diffusely edematous and infiltrated by a small number of lymphocytes and monocytes. The outer medullary vasa recta often contain large numbers of nucleated circulating cells including lymphocytes and monocytes, both

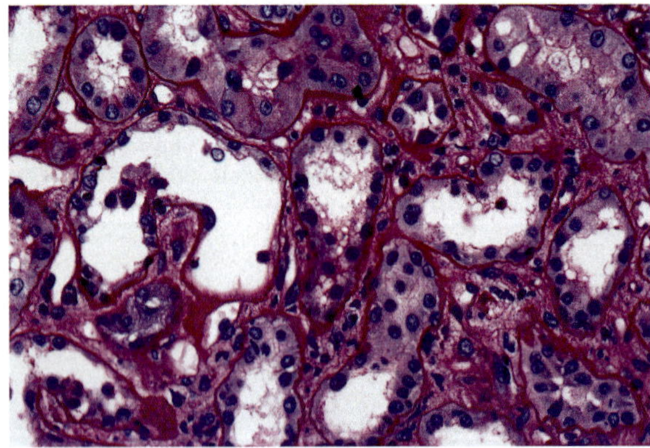

FIGURE 15.1. Tubular cells are flattened and many proximal cells lack brush border staining; lumina are relatively dilated [periodic acid-schiff (PAS) stain].

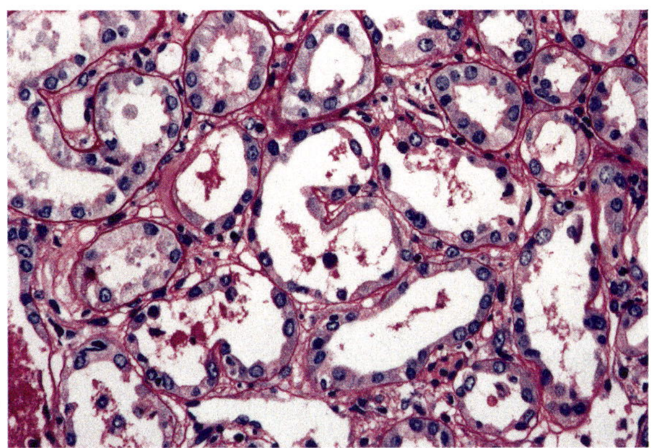

FIGURE 15.2. One tubule contains cells and debris in lumen and is incompletely lined by epithelium (PAS stain).

mature and immature forms, and granulocyte precursors. These cells are in greater concentrations in the vasa recta than in other renal vascular beds. The glomerular capillary tufts are usually unaltered. However, there are several reasonably common abnormalities: there may be some degree of capillary collapse and dilatation of Bowman's space. Additionally, tubular metaplasia ("tubularization") of parietal epithelial cells may be evident in recovery. Solez and colleagues (5) assessed these morphologic changes as to their frequency in active renal failure, recovery phase, and normal controls. In their landmark study, they noted that the following were more common in biopsies from patients with renal failure: vasa recta leukocyte accumulation, tubular cell necrosis, regeneration (mitotic figures), dilatation of Bowman's spaces, loss of brush border staining, tubular casts, and interstitial edema and inflammation. However, only cellular necrosis and loss of brush border staining distinguished biopsies from patients with acute renal failure from those of patients in recovery from renal failure.

Electron Microscopy

Ultrastructural observations have indicated a reduction in brush border formation for most proximal tubules; this ranges from slight to almost complete loss of microvilli. There is also simplification of basolateral cell surfaces. Overt necrosis is also noted. Disintegration of cells, characterized by extreme lucency of cytoplasm together with disruption of plasma membrane, nuclear membrane, or organelles, may affect single cells, with only minor abnormalities to neighboring cells. Apoptosis, characterized by condensation and increased density of cytoplasm and closely aggregated organelles, dilated vacuoles, cisternae and mitochondria, and folding of nuclear membrane with clumped chromatin, affects single cells, and is increased compared to normal. The above-mentioned nonreplacement phenomenon is identified as a defect in epithelial lining corresponding to loss of a single cell; the intact basement membrane may be covered by a thin projection of cytoplasm from an adjacent cell.

Toxic Acute Tubular Necrosis

Pathologic Findings

The basic morphologic findings in toxic ATN, rarely observed today, are best illustrated in mercuric chloride poisoning. At 3 days following exposure, there is extensive necrosis of cells of the proximal convoluted tubules; the necrotic cells are partially desquamated and the lumina are filled with cellular debris. At 7 to 9 days, most of the luminal contents are no longer present in the proximal tubules but are in more distal parts of the nephron. The proximal tubules are dilated and lined by flattened and basophilic cells with numerous mitotic figures. At 2 weeks, the proximal tubules are lined by cuboidal epithelium; tubular calcifications are not infrequent. In general, tubular basement membranes are intact, and interstitial edema with a variable mononuclear leukocytic infiltrate is evident. This sequence of events is reasonably constant for other agents, although the degree of overt necrosis rarely achieves that of mercuric chloride. There are some morphologic features that are reasonably characteristic of certain toxins; they may be observed by light or electron microscopy depending on the poison. For example, gentamicin may result in ultrastructurally defined myeloid bodies (lysosomes with phospholipid), lead is characterized by intranuclear inclusions (consisting of lead and lead-binding protein) as is bismuth, and gold accumulates in lysosomes in tubular cells as dense filamentous structures (aureosomes).

Etiology/Pathogenesis

The pathogenesis of acute renal failure in ATN has been studied extensively and, at least in humans, no clear, coherent, and universally acceptable explanation exists at present. Increased tubular permeability to glomerular filtrate (backleak) through an injured tubular wall (cells) probably plays a role in more severe ischemic and toxic ATN, but likely is unimportant in mild to moderate acute renal failure. Tubule obstruction, because of luminal casts, debris, cells, and/or crystals, may have some role in altering renal function (6). Reduction in renal cortical and glomerular blood flow is documented and is responsible for the gross autopsy findings of cortical pallor. Its mechanism may be related to vasoconstrictive humoral factors. Medullary blood flow reduction has also been documented, especially at the corticomedullary junction, affecting juxtamedullary nephrons. This regional hypoxia could explain the apparent susceptibility of the straight portion of the proximal tubule (S3) to ischemia; the medullary thick ascending limb may also be affected similarly. Tubuloglomerular feedback activation is implicated in some phases of acute renal failure, although its extent and the importance of vasoactive substances are not clarified. Rosen, Brezis, and coworkers (7,8), in a series of studies on experimentally induced acute renal failure, documented the regular occurrence of necrosis of cells of the thick ascending limb of Henle (TALH). The lesions affected only a few cells of this portion of the nephron and therefore are often difficult to detect in many biopsies unless sufficient medullary tissue is available. Because the cells of TALH are involved with feedback control of glomerular filtration and with production of Tamm-Horsfall protein as casts that may obstruct the nephron, injury to these cells may well be directly responsible for acute renal failure. These investigators have maintained that necrosis of thick ascending limb cells is the primary and, indeed, pathophysiologically important lesion in ATN with acute renal failure. The other changes of cells in different segments of the nephron are viewed, perhaps correctly so, as secondary lesions. The work of Brezis, Rosen, and colleagues points out the importance of reduced renal blood flow to the inner strip of the medulla and the thick ascending limb of Henle in animals and suggests its applicability to human acute renal failure, including the lesion known as "lower nephron nephrosis."

References

1. Kashgarian M. Acute tubular necrosis and ischemic renal injury. In: Jennette JC, Olson JL, Schwartz MM, Silva FG, eds. Heptinstall's Pathology of the Kidney, 5th ed. Philadelphia: Lippincott-Raven, 1998:863–889.
2. Olsen S, Solez K. Acute tubular necrosis and toxic renal injury. In: Tisher CC, Brenner BM, eds. Renal Pathology with Clinical and Functional Correlations, 2nd ed. Philadelphia: Lippincott, 1994:769–809.
3. Thadhani R, Pascual M, Bonventre JV. Acute renal failure. N Engl J Med 334:1448–1460, 1996.
4. Nadasdy T, Racusen LC. Renal injury caused by therapeutic and diagnostic agents and abuse of analgesics and narcotics. In: Jennette JC, Olson JL, Schwartz MM, Silva FG, eds. Heptinstall's Pathology of the Kidney, 5th ed. Philadelphia: Lippincott-Raven, 1998:811–862.
5. Solez K, Morel-Maroger L, Sraer JD. The morphology of "acute tubular necrosis" in man: analysis of 57 renal biopsies and a comparison with the glycerol model. Medicine 58:362–376, 1979.
6. Molitoris BA, Marrs J. The role of cell adhesion molecules in ischemic renal failure. Am J Med 106:583–592, 1999.
7. Brezis M, Rosen S. Hypoxia of the renal medulla—its implications for disease. N Engl J Med 332:647–655, 1995.
8. Rosen S, Heyman SN. Difficulties in understanding human "acute tubular necrosis": limited data and flawed animal models. Kidney Int 60:1220–1224, 2001.

Section VII
Plasma Cell Dyscrasias and Associated Renal Diseases

Introduction

There are many renal lesions that occur in the plasma cell dyscrasias; some are the result of deposition or accumulation of the abnormal immunoglobulin, usually the light chain component, in various locations, whereas others are infectious and metabolic complications of the underlying malignancy. This section discusses the major paraprotein-induced lesions. Each has distinct pathologic features and different pathogenic mechanisms. Clinical findings are variable, although the cast nephropathy general presents with acute renal failure while the deposition diseases present with glomerular proteinuria. Any of the lesions may be the initial manifestation of the plasma cell dyscrasia or may be manifested in a patient already known to have a plasma cell dyscrasia (1).

16
Bence Jones Cast Nephropathy

Arthur H. Cohen

Clinical Presentation

Patients with Bence Jones cast nephropathy usually present with acute renal failure (less commonly with chronic renal failure) and Bence Jones proteinuria. It has been known for many years that intravenous radiocontrast media, dehydration, infections, and the use of nonsteroidal antiinflammatory drugs may induce the precipitation of renal tubular light chain casts and result in acute renal failure, which is reversible in only a small percent of affected patients. A less common manner of presentation is the acquired Fanconi syndrome. This is most often associated with intracellular crystals in plasma cells and tubular cells; the crystals represent the abnormal light chain (2,3).

Pathologic Findings

Light Microscopy

Bence Jones cast nephropathy is characterized by prominent casts in renal tubules; the casts are usually large and "brittle," have fracture lines or are broken into many fragments often with geometric shapes, and are surrounded by tubular epithelium, neutrophils, and typically and diagnostically by multinucleated giant cells of foreign-body type (Fig. 16.1). While they are more common in distal tubules, the casts may be formed in any segment of the nephron, including Bowman's space. The casts have reasonably typical tinctorial properties: periodic acid-Schiff (PAS) negative, brightly eosinophilic, fuchsinophilic with Masson's trichrome and, infrequently, Congo red positive. The staining is not always uniform within the same cast or among all casts in the same kidney, but the above colors are most typical. The casts may be lamellated, contain crystals of a variety of shapes, and, rarely at the periphery have a spicular appearance. There are reasonably constant abnormalities in tubular epithelium; proximal cells often contain numerous uniform cytoplasmic vacuoles. Cells of all tubular

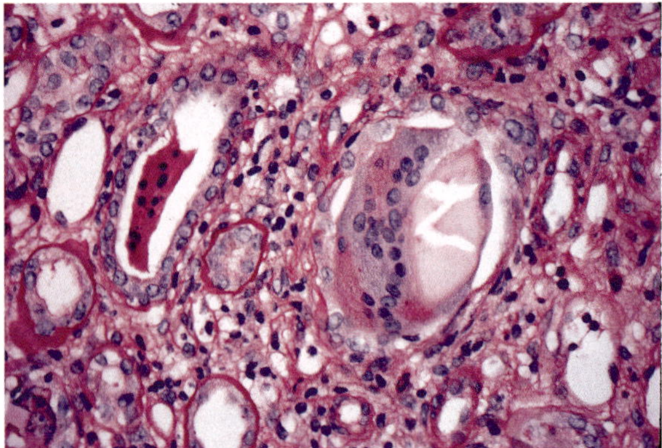

Figure 16.1. Bence Jones (light chain)cast nephropathy with a tubule containing a pale-staining cast surrounded by a multinucleated giant cell. In contrast, casts composed primarily of Tamm-Horsfall protein are periodic acid-Schiff (PAS) positive (PAS stain).

segments may be necrotic and sloughed into lumina, where they may be adherent to the edges of the casts. Tubular basement membranes are discontinuous, thereby allowing free communication between the interstitium and the tubular lumina; it is through these gaps that monocytes and other inflammatory cells migrate from the interstitium. The adjacent interstitium is edematous and often infiltrated by monocytes and lymphocyte (1–4). This constellation of light microscopic abnormalities, especially the morphology and tinctorial properties of the casts and the surrounding giant cells, is sufficiently distinctive to be diagnostic of multiple myeloma. Indeed, it is not unusual for the renal biopsy to be the first test indicative of myeloma in a patient who presents with acute renal failure of seemingly unknown origin (5).

Immunohistochemistry

The composition of the casts has been determined by immunohistochemistry. Most investigators have documented that they consist exclusively or primarily of the abnormal light chain (1,2). Depending on many factors, Tamm-Horsfall protein and the other light chain may also be part of the casts. Many other plasma proteins may also be present. When the other proteins are present, they are usually in a staining intensity less than the abnormal light chain. By immunofluorescence, it is possible to detect Tamm-Horsfall protein in glomerular urinary spaces, a finding that is indicative of obstruction (either intrarenal or extrarenal) of urine with retrograde flow in the nephron. The ultrastructural appearance of the casts is quite variable, although the basic structure is of a mass of deeply electron-dense material. The casts may be homogeneous, finely or coarsely granular, and may incorporate cytoplasmic debris (4).

Etiology/Pathogenesis

The pathogenesis of cast nephropathy has been partially elucidated, although there are still many unanswered questions. The free abnormal light chain is freely filtered by the glomerulus and, for unclear reasons either because of quantity or quality, it is toxic to tubular epithelium (proximal and distal). Furthermore, in the distal nephron (thick ascending limb of Henle), Bence Jones protein coprecipitates with Tamm-Horsfall protein, thus forming casts (6). It is likely that Bence Jones protein alone can also precipitate in tubules, thereby explaining the presence of the casts in the proximal nephron. It is also likely that a combination of direct damage to tubular cells (tubular necrosis), which is associated with tubular basement membrane breaks, and the physical effects of the geometrically shaped casts leads to tubular wall disruption and migration of monocytes into tubules to surround casts and form multinucleated giant cells. Because of the large size of the casts, they likely obstruct the nephron in which they are formed. Thus, it appears that renal impairment in Bence Jones cast nephropathy is the result of tubular necrosis, interstitial inflammation, and nephron obstruction (1,4).

Investigators during the last decade or so have sought to identify that which confers "nephrotoxicity" on light chains; in addition, as there are several light chain–induced renal lesions, investigations to ascertain why a particular light chain will produce one lesion rather than another are underway. It is likely that host factors are not of prime importance; the intrinsic physical or chemical properties of light chains are thought to be of greatest significance. However, despite initial evidence linking light chain isoelectric point, molecular weight, degree of polymerization, and size, among others, to the development of this or the other light chain–induced renal lesions, at the present time no property of monoclonal light chains has been identified to explain their nephrotoxic potential (2,3). It is of interest to note, however, that monoclonal light chains from humans with specific light chain–induced lesions (cast nephropathy, light chain deposit disease, amyloid), when injected into mice, induced the same renal abnormality as in humans as elegantly documented by Solomon and colleagues (7) in 1991.

References

1. Cohen AH. The kidney in plasma cell dyscrasias: Bence Jones cast nephropathy and light chain deposit disease. Am J Kidney Dis 32:529–532, 1998.
2. Schwartz MM. The dysproteinemias and amyloidosis. In: Jennette JC, Olson JL, Schwartz MM, Silva FG, eds. Heptinstall's Pathology of the Kidney, 5th ed. Philadelphia: Lippincott-Raven, 1998:1321.
3. Striker LJM-M, Preudhomme JL, D'Amico G, Striker GE. Monoclonal gammopathies, mixed cryoglobulinemias, and lymphomas. In: Tisher CC, Brenner BM, eds. Renal Pathology with Clinical and Functional Correlations, 2nd ed. Philadelphia: JB Lippincott, 1994:1442.

4. Cohen AH, Border WA. Myeloma kidney; an immunomorphogenetic study of renal biopsies. Lab Invest 42:248, 1980.
5. Border WA, Cohen AH. Renal biopsy diagnosis of clinically silent multiple myeloma. Ann Intern Med 93:43–46, 1980.
6. Huang ZQ, Sanders PW. Localization of a single binding site for immunoglobulin light chains on human Tamm-Horsfall glycoprotein. J Clin Invest 99:732–736, 1997.
7. Solomon A, Weiss DT, Kattine AA. Nephrotoxic potentials of Bence Jones proteins. N Engl J Med 324:1845–1851, 1991.

17 Monoclonal Immunoglobulin Deposition Disease

Arthur H. Cohen

Introduction/Clinical Setting

Patients with plasma cell dyscrasias may have other forms of renal disease than light chain cast nephropathy. These include the closely related systemic disorders amyloidosis (AL type) and light chain deposit disease (1–7). In the kidneys, although both of these conditions clinically and pathologically affect primarily glomeruli, there is important and often constant involvement of tubular basement membranes, interstitium, and arteries. On rare occasions, the intact monoclonal protein (light and heavy chains) or heavy chain alone may deposit in renal basement membranes and systemically. Consequently, these disorders, originally considered solely of abnormal light chain pathogenesis and termed by some as light chain deposit diseases or nephropathies, are more correctly termed and thought of as monoclonal immunoglobulin deposition diseases (5). Evaluation of immunoglobulin synthesis by bone marrow cells has determined incomplete light chains and/or heavy chain fragments (8).

Light Chain Deposition Disease/Heavy Chain Deposition Disease

Light chain deposit disease is characterized by the nonimmune deposition of a monoclonal light chain in all renal basement membranes as well as the glomerular mesangium. Renal involvement is part of a systemic disease, for virtually all other organs and tissues are also the sites of light chain deposits. The kidneys are the most important organs involved in terms of clinical manifestations, although some patients can develop significant and fatal cardiac lesions (1–3,5).

Pathologic Findings

Light Microscopy

Light chain deposit disease can have many of the light microscopic morphologic features of diabetic nephropathy, especially because of the nodular glomerular lesions and capillary microaneurysms (2,3,9,10).

The light microscopic appearance of glomeruli was initially emphasized as a nodular glomerulopathy with features virtually indistinguishable from nodular diabetic glomerulosclerosis (Fig. 17.1); however, it has become apparent that there is a large spectrum of glomerular morphologies including normal glomeruli, diffuse widening of mesangium, crescents, etc. The tubular basement membrane deposits often result in the light microscopic appreciation of thickened tubular basement membranes. Careful high magnification examination of periodic acid-Schiff (PAS)-stained sections may indicate a slightly lighter staining band external to the normal basement membrane (1).

Heavy chain deposition disease is characterized by the nonimmunologic binding of an abnormal heavy chain, most commonly immunoglobulin G (IgG), to all basement membranes (8,10). The morphologic aspects differ from light chain deposit disease in that the glomerular structure is almost always nodular. However, glomerular hypercellularity mimicking membranoproliferative or other proliferative glomerulonephritis may be the dominant morphology (11,12).

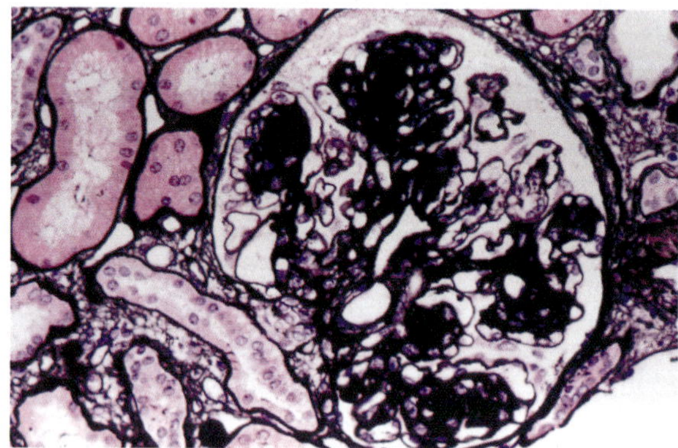

FIGURE 17.1. Light chain deposition disease with glomerulus with nodular mesangium. This appearance is similar to diabetic nodular glomerulosclerosis (Jones silver stain).

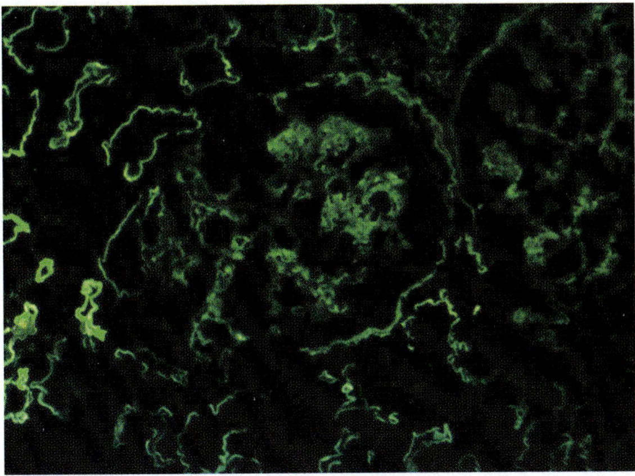

FIGURE 17.2. Light chain deposition disease with linear staining of all renal basement membranes and mesangial regions of the glomeruli (kappa immunofluorescence).

Immunofluorescence Microscopy

These disorders require immunofluorescence evaluation of tissue sections, for the diagnosis rests on documenting a single light and/or heavy chain in the tissue basement membranes. Thus, the diagnosis of this deposition disease can be made only with the routine use of immunofluorescence; one cannot rely on the glomerular morphology to dictate when to evaluate the biopsy with antibodies to the light chains. Immunofluorescence shows monoclonal prominent staining along the tubular and glomerular basement membranes (Fig. 17.2). In the absence of tissue for immunofluorescence, documentation of ultrastructurally defined deposits when present (see below) should serve as a strong indication of light chains. In heavy chain deposition disease, when IgG3 is the paraprotein, complement is also deposited with associated hypocomplementemia (13).

Electron Microscopy

The ultrastructural manifestations of the light chain deposits are of clustered punctate dense deposits external to tubular and within vascular basement membranes (2,3). Deposits in the glomerular basement membranes are similar (Fig. 17.3), whereas they are variably evident in the mesangium. However, there may be no electron microscopic counterpart of the immunofluorescence deposition (1).

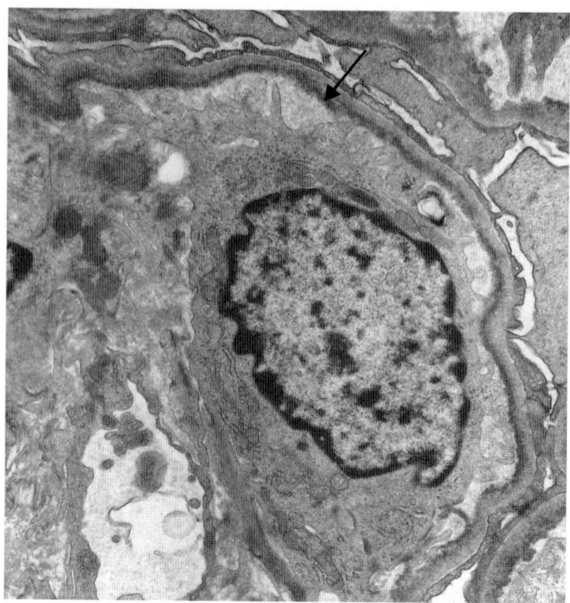

FIGURE 17.3. Light chain deposition disease with continuous granular density in glomerular basement membrane (arrow) (electron microscopy).

Etiology/Pathogenesis

Clinically, this renal lesion presents with heavy proteinuria (both light chain and larger plasma proteins), renal insufficiency, and sometimes hypertension. Approximately 50% of the patients have overt myeloma; the rest have either plasmacytosis or no evidence of increased plasma cells (1–3,7). In this last instance, there is increased immunoglobulin synthesis with excess light chain production. Therapy may result in the disappearance of nodules and improvement of renal function (14).

References

1. Cohen AH. The kidney in plasma cell dyscrasias: Bence Jones cast nephropathy and light chain deposit disease. Am J Kidney Dis 32:529–532, 1998.
2. Schwartz MM. The dysproteinemias and amyloidosis. In: Jennette JC, Olson JL, Schwartz MM, Silva FG, eds. Heptinstall's Pathology of the Kidney, 5th ed. Philadelphia: Lippincott-Raven, 1998:1321.
3. Striker LJM-M, Preudhomme JL, D'Amico G, Striker GE. Monoclonal gammopathies, mixed cryoglobulinemias, and lymphomas. In: Tisher CC, Brenner BM, eds. Renal Pathology with Clinical and Functional Correlations, 2nd ed. Philadelphia: JB Lippincott, 1994:1442.

4. Solomon A, Weiss DT, Kattine AA. Nephrotoxic potentials of Bence Jones proteins. N Engl J Med 324:1845–1851, 1991.
5. Buxbaum JN, Chuba JV, Hellman GC, Solomon A, Gallo GR. Monoclonal immunoglobulin deposition disease: light chain and light and heavy chain deposition diseases and their relationship to light chain amyloidosis: clinical features, immunopathology, and molecular analysis. Ann Intern Med 112:455–464, 1990.
6. Montseny JJ, Kleinknecht D, Meyrier A, et al. Long-term outcome according to renal histological lesions in 118 patients with monoclonal gammopathies. Nephrol Dial Transplant 13:1438–1445, 1998.
7. Preudhomme J-L, Aucouturier P, Touchard G, et al. Monoclonal immunoglobulin deposition disease (Randall type): relationship with structural abnormalities of immunoglobulin chains. Kidney Int 46:965–972, 1994.
8. Buxbaum JN. Abnormal immunoglobulin synthesis in monoclonal immunoglobulin light chain and light and heavy chain deposition disease. Amyloid 8:84–93, 2001.
9. Sinniah R, Cohen AH. Glomerular capillary aneurysms in light chain nephropathy: an ultrastructural proposal of pathogenesis. Am J Pathol 118:298–305, 1985.
10. Lin J, Markowitz GS, Valeri AM, et al. Renal monoclonal immunoglobulin deposition disease: the disease spectrum. J Am Soc Nephrol 12:1482–1492, 2001.
11. Nasr SH, Markowitz GS, Stokes MB, et al. Proliferative glomerulonephritis with monoclonal IgG deposits: a distinct entity mimicking immune-complex glomerulonephritis. Kidney Int 65:85–96, 2004.
12. Vedder AC, Weening JJ, Krediet RT. Intracapillary proliferative glomerulonephritis due to heavy chain deposition disease. Nephrol Dial Transplant 19:1302–1304, 2004.
13. Soma J, Sato K, Sakuma T, et al. Immunoglobulin gamma-3-heavy-chain deposition disease: report of a case and relationship with hypocomplementemia. Am J Kidney Dis 43:E10–16, 2004.
14. Komatsuda A, Wakui H, Ohtani H, et al. Disappearance of nodular mesangial lesions in a patient with light chain nephropathy after long-term chemotherapy. Am J Kidney Dis 35:E9, 2000.

18
Amyloidosis

Arthur H. Cohen

Introduction/Clinical Setting

Amyloidosis (AL type) is conceptually similar to light chain deposit disease in many respects (1). It represents the systemic deposition of a structurally altered light and/or heavy chain and is more common than light chain deposit disease. Amyloid may also be due to deposition of other proteins that form beta-pleated sheets. Most patients with glomerular amyloid present with heavy proteinuria and approximately 50% have concurrent renal insufficiency. Interstitial or vascular (nonglomerular) amyloid morphologically is similar to amyloid in other locations; in the absence of glomerular amyloid, its detection requires a reasonably high level of suspicion on the part of the pathologist. Isolated interstitial amyloid is usually manifested by some degree of renal insufficiency; "pure" vascular amyloid may be clinically silent or may be associated with renal functional impairment.

Pathologic Findings

Light Microscopy

Amyloid appears as amorphous acellular, pale eosinophilic material in the mesangium and extending out to glomerular capillary walls in some patients (Fig. 18.1). The capillary wall deposits may appear as silverpositive fringe-like projections, longer than those seen in membranous glomerulopathy. Arterioles and arteries frequently show amyloid deposits as well. The renal pathologic features of other varieties of amyloid (e.g., AA, hereditary forms, etc.) are virtually identical in most respects to AL amyloid (1,2). Specific diagnosis is made by positive Congo red stain, with apple green birefringence under polarized light (Fig. 18.2).

Immunofluorescence Microscopy

When amyloid is due to monoclonal AL, immunofluorescence may show smudgy positivity in affected areas for the responsible light chain.

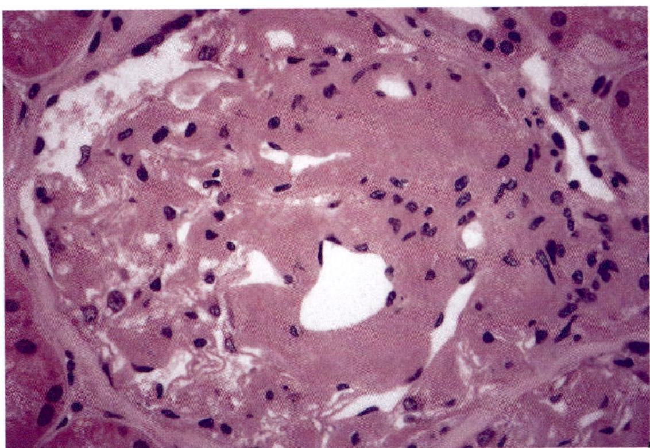

FIGURE 18.1. Amyloid with glomerulus and arteriole infiltrated by homogeneous acellular material replacing normal structures [periodic acid-Schiff (PAS) stain].

Lambda light chain more commonly gives rise to amyloid than does kappa. Other types of amyloid do not stain for light chains by immunofluorescence, but may be detected by immunohistochemistry, with antibodies for specific amyloidogenic proteins such as AA.

Electron Microscopy

Randomly arranged fibrils, 10 to 12 nm, are present in extracellular sites in affected arterioles and arteries, mesangial areas, often infiltrating GBMs, and occasionally in the interstitium (Fig. 18.3).

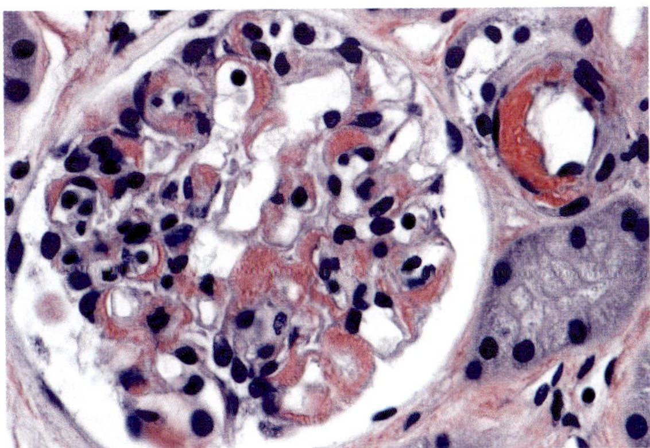

FIGURE 18.2. Congo red stain disclosing the abnormal material to stain positively, diagnostic of amyloid.

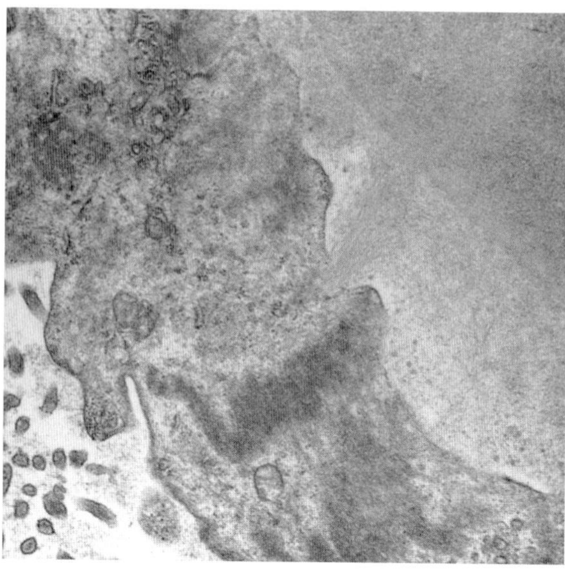

FIGURE 18.3. The abnormal material in amyloid is composed of numerous fine fibrils seen on electron microscopy.

Etiology/Pathogenesis

Amyloid is composed of insoluble poorly degradable 10-nm fibrils that are commonly haphazardly arranged in basement membranes and walls of all types of vessels and in the interstitium around capillaries. In the kidneys, the glomeruli are usually initially involved and almost always represent the most important component affected. In AL, the abnormal light chain (usually lambda VI subtype) is transformed into a beta-pleated sheet structure, which is responsible for the morphologic, optical, and tinctorial properties of amyloid. On rare occasions, amyloid may be composed solely of an monoclonal heavy chain (3–5). Although some clinical and laboratory findings, including a negative family history, may appear to point to AL amyloid, a study documented amyloidogenic gene mutations indicating a hereditary form of amyloid in 10% of such patients (6). In addition, one study documented lack of sensitivity in using immunofluorescence as a means of identifying either light chain as the amyloid-producing protein (7). This suggests that, in patients with amyloid in which AA is not documented and protein/light chain and bone marrow confirmation of AL amyloid is lacking, genetic causes of amyloid be considered. Work by Herrera et al concerning interaction between abnormal light chains and cultured mesangial cells indicates that the ability of the light chain to be internalized by the cell may be an important factor in the development of amyloid rather than light chain deposition disease. Further, cast-producing light chains had no effect on mesangial cells (8).

Similar to light chain deposit disease, patients with AL amyloid may have overt myeloma or only a slight plasmacytosis. Roughly 80% do not have myeloma; conversely, amyloid occurs in approximately 7% to 10% of patients with myeloma. Although these light chain-induced renal lesions have been presented here as isolated entities, the coexistence of any two or even all three is well known (1,2).

References

1. Schwartz MM. The dysproteinemias and amyloidosis. In: Jennette JC, Olson JL, Schwartz MM, Silva FG, eds. Heptinstall's Pathology of the Kidney, 5th ed. Philadelphia: Lippincott-Raven, 1998:1321.
2. Striker LJM-M, Preudhomme JL, D'Amico G, Striker GE. Monoclonal gammopathies, mixed cryoglobulinemias, and lymphomas. In: Tisher CC, Brenner BM, eds. Renal Pathology with Clinical and Functional Correlations, 2nd ed. Philadelphia: JB Lippincott, 1994:1442.
3. Mai HL, Sheikh-Hamad D, Herrera GA, Gu X, Truong LD. Immunoglobulin heavy chain can be amyloidogenic: morphologic characterization including immunoelectron microscopy. Am J Surg Pathol 27:541–545, 2003.
4. Copeland JN, Kouides PA, Grieff M, Nadasdy T. Metachronous development of nonamyloidogenic lambda night chain deposition disease and IgG heavy chain amyloidosis in the same patient. Am J Surg Pathol 27:1477–1482, 2003.
5. Yazaki M, Fushimi T, Tokuda T, et al. A patient with severe renal amyloidosis associated with an immunoglobulin gamma-heavy chain fragment. Am J Kidney Dis 43:e23–28, 2004.
6. Lachmann HJ, Booth DR, Booth SE, et al. Misdiagnosis of hereditary amyloidosis as AL (primary) amyloidosis. N Engl J Med 346:1786–1791, 2002.
7. Novak L, Cook WJ, Herrera GA, Sanders PW. AL-amyloidosis is underdiagnosed in renal biopsies. Nephrol Dial Transplant 19:3050–3053, 2004.
8. Keeling J, Teng J, Herrera GA. Al-amyloidosis and light chain deposition disease light chains induce divergent transformations of human mesangial cells. Lab Invest 84:1322–1338, 2004.

19
Other Diseases with Organized Deposits

Arthur H. Cohen

Fibrillary Glomerulonephritis

Pathologic Findings

Other abnormal substances may infiltrate the glomeruli and cause significant dysfunction. Perhaps among the more important of these is the lesion known as fibrillary glomerulonephritis (Fig. 19.1) (1–3). The light microscopy of glomeruli indicates variable increase in mesangial cellularity and irregularly thickened capillary walls. Crescents may be present (1,4). Immunofluorescence is positive, with coarse linear/confluent granular immunoglobulin G (IgG), C3, and one or both light chains. This disorder is ultrastructurally defined and is characterized by the accumulation of fibrils that are roughly 10 to 20 nm in diameter and are throughout the mesangial matrix and basement membranes in a manner very similar to amyloid (1). Indeed, the fibrils bear striking similarity to amyloid. In contrast, however, the infiltrate is Congo red negative, unlike amyloid (5).

Extraglomerular and extrarenal involvement is rare (6,7). The typical clinical presentation is of heavy proteinuria with hematuria, hypertension, and some degree of renal insufficiency. Serologic studies are negative or noncontributory, although some patients may have a positive antinuclear antibody (ANA). This disorder runs a chronic course with advanced renal insufficiency requiring renal replacement therapy in approximately 40%. The nature if the fibrils is not known; one report described a circulating cryoprecipitated factor composed of immunoglobulins, light chains, and fibronectin (3). The disease not infrequently recurs in the transplant (8,9). A comparison between amyloid and fibrillary glomerulonephritis is indicated in Table 19.1.

Immunotactoid Glomerulopathy

Another disorder with peculiar ultrastructural features is known as immunotactoid glomerulopathy (Fig. 19.2) (1,4,10). The light microscopic appearance of glomeruli is typically of a membranoproliferative

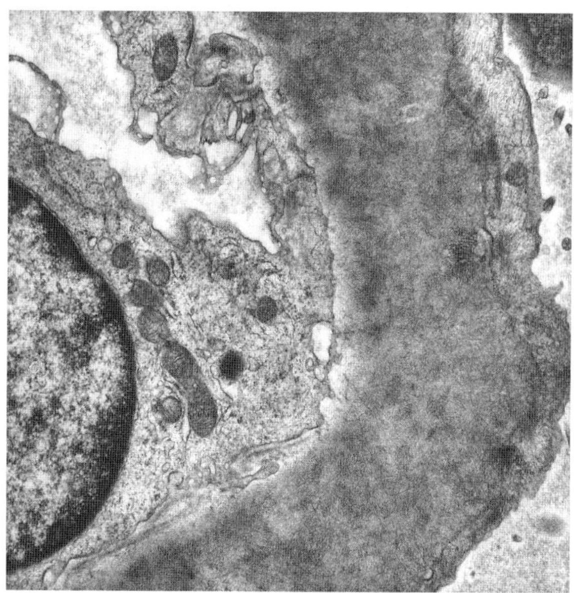

FIGURE 19.1. Fibrillary glomerulonephritis; there are numerous randomly arranged fine fibrils permeating the basement membrane (electron microscopy).

glomerulonephritis type I pattern. Immunofluorescence microscopy discloses granular capillary wall deposits of IgG, complement, and one or both light chains. In this entity, glomerular immune (electron-dense) deposits are composed of numerous coarse hollow-cored fibrils (immunotactoids) ranging in thickness from approximately 20 to 80nm. Patients present with heavy proteinuria and hematuria; approximately 50% have been found to have a concurrent or subsequently developing lymphoproliferative disease (1,11).

TABLE 19.1. Features of amyloid and fibrillary glomerulonephritis (GN)

Amyloid	Fibrillary GN
Fibrils 10–12nm	Fibrils 10–20nm
Extraglomerular renal involvement—vessels, interstitium, etc.	Rare extraglomerular renal involvement
Extrarenal involvement common	Extrarenal involvement rare
Congo red positive	Congo red negative

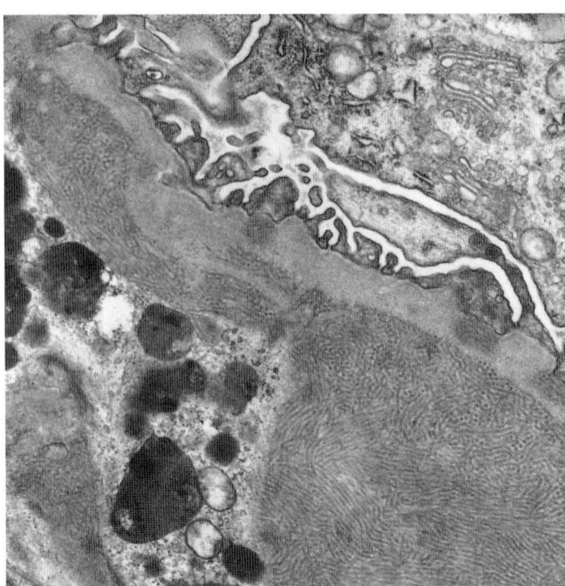

FIGURE 19.2. Immunotactoid glomerulopathy; the large subendothelial deposit is composed of many hollow-cored tubular structures, some of which are in cross section (electron microscopy).

Clinical Correlations

Until recently, a controversy existed concerning these two diseases (1,12,13). Some investigators consider them to be the same entity based on clinical presentation and course as well as ultrastructural features that are thought to represent structural manifestations of abnormal protein deposits. Other investigators, however, deem these disorders to be completely separate and distinct entities that happen to be diagnosed on the basis of ultrastructural abnormalities. Studies by Bridoux et al (11) and Rosenstock et al (4) have quite convincingly demonstrated that the distinct pathologic features are associated with distinct clinical manifestations and significance. Most important is the tight link between immunotactoid glomerulopathy and lymphoproliferative disorders (11).

References

1. Fogo A, Qureshi N, Horn RG. Morphologic and clinical features of fibrillary glomerulonephritis versus immunotactoid glomerulopathy. Am J Kidney Dis 22:367–377, 1993.
2. Ferrario F, Schiaffino E, Boeri R. Fibrillary and immunotactoid glomerulopathies. Ren Fail 20:801–808, 1998.

3. Rostagno A, Vidal R, Kumar A, et al. Fibrillary glomerulonephritis related to serum fibrillar immunoglobulin-fibronectin complexes. Am J Kidney Dis 28:676–684, 1996.
4. Rosenstock JL, Markowitz GS, Valeri AM, Sacchi G, Appel GB, D'Agati VD. Fibrillary and immunotactoid glomerulonephritis: distinct entities with different clinical and pathologic features. Kidney Int 63:1450–1461, 2003.
5. Rosenman E, Eliakim M. Nephrotic syndrome associated with amyloid-like glomerular deposits. Nephron 18:301–308, 1997.
6. Adeya OA, Sethi S, Rennke HG. Fibrillary glomerulonephritis: a report of 2 cases with extensive glomerular and tubular deposits. Hum Pathol 32:660–663, 2001.
7. Masson RG, Rennke HG, Gottlieb MN. Pulmonary hemorrhage in a patient with fibrillary glomerulonephritis. N Engl J Med 326:3639, 1992.
8. Pronovost PH, Brady HR, Gunning ME, Espinoza O, Rennke HG. Clinical features, predictors of disease progression and results of renal transplantation in fibrillary/immunotactoid glomerulopathy. Nephrol Dial Transplant 11:837–842, 1996.
9. Samaniego M, Nadasdy GM, Laszik Z, Nadasdy T. Outcome of renal transplantation in fibrillary glomerulonephritis. Clin Nephrol 55:159–166, 2001.
10. Korbet SM, Schwartz MM, Lewis EJ. Immunotactoid glomerulopathy. Am J Kidney Dis 17:247–257, 1991.
11. Bridoux F, Hugue V, Coldefy O, et al. Fibrillary glomerulonephritis and immunotactoid (microtubular) glomerulopathy are associated with distinct immunologic features. Kidney Int 62:1764–1775, 2002.
12. Schwartz MM. Immunotactoid glomerulopathy. The case for Occam's razor. Am J Kidney Dis 22:446–447, 1993.
13. Korbet SM, Schwartz MM, Lewis EJ. The fibrillary glomerulopathies. Am J Kidney Dis 23:751–765, 1994.

Section VIII
Renal Transplant Pathology

20
Allograft Rejection

Robert B. Colvin

The renal transplant biopsy remains the gold standard for the diagnosis of episodes of graft dysfunction that occur in 10% to 30% of patients after transplantation. In a prospective trial at the Massachusetts General Hospital, the biopsy diagnosis changed the patient management as based on the prebiopsy clinical diagnosis in 42% of graft dysfunction episodes (39% in the first month, 56% in the first year, and 39% after 1 year); in 19% unnecessary immunosuppression was avoided (1). The present review is updated from prior publications by the author (2,3). My preferred pathologic classification of the diseases of renal allografts is given in Table 20.1.

Acute Cellular Rejection (ACR)

Introduction/Clinical Setting

Acute cellular rejection is the common form of rejection, mediated by T cells, that develops classically 1 to 6 weeks after transplantation, but may erupt at any time, even after many years. The typical clinical presentation is a rising serum creatinine over a few days, accompanied by weight gain and sometimes fever and graft tenderness.

Pathologic Findings

Light Microscopy

The sites of acute cellular rejection are the interstitium, tubules, endothelium, and glomeruli. They may be involved separately or in combination.

The characteristic microscopic feature of type I rejection is a pleomorphic interstitial infiltrate of activated lymphocytes and monocytes, accompanied by interstitial edema and tubular injury. The cells invade tubules ("tubulitis") and infiltrate the cortex (10–25% in the Banff system is considered suspicious for rejection and >25% is rejection) (Fig. 20.1).

TABLE 20.1. Pathologic classification of renal allograft lesions

I. Immunologic rejection
  A. Acute cellular rejection (ACR)
    1. Tubulo-interstitial (CCTT/Banff type I + Banff suspicious)
    2. Vascular (endothelialitis) (CCTT/Banff type II)
    3. Glomerular (acute allograft glomerulopathy) (No CCTT/Banff type)
  B. Acute humoral rejection (AHR) (termed hyperacute rejection when in first 24 hours)
    1. Acute tubular injury [C4d^{+} peritubular capillaries PTCs; new category]
    2. Capillary inflammation (C4d^{+} PTCs; new category)
    3. Arterial fibrinoid necrosis (previously CCTT/Banff type III)
  C. Chronic allograft rejection: Arterial intimal thickening, glomerulopathy and/or interstitial fibrosis and tubular atrophy with immunologic activity
    a. Chronic active humoral rejection (C4d^{+})
    b. Chronic active cellular rejection (T cells in lesions)
  D. Non–human leukocyte antigen (HLA) alloantibody-mediated renal diseases
    1. De novo membranous glomerulonephritis
    2. Anti–glomerular basement membrane (GBM) disease (in Alport's syndrome)
    3. Anti–tubular basement membrane (TBM) disease
II. Nonrejection injury
  A. Acute ischemic injury (ATN)
  B. Perfusion injury
  C. Calcineurin inhibitor nephrotoxicity (cyclosporine, tacrolimus)
    1. Acute
      a. Functional
      b. Tubular
      c. Vascular
    2. Thrombotic microangiopathy
    3. Chronic
      a. Tubulo-interstitial
      b. Vascular (hyalinosis)
  D. Other Drug Toxicity
    1. OKT3
    2. Rapamycin
  E. Major artery/vein thrombosis
  F. Renal artery stenosis
  G. Obstruction
  H. Infection (viral, bacterial, fungal)
  I. Acute tubulo-interstitial nephritis (drug allergy)
  J. De novo glomerular disease
    1. Focal segmental glomerular sclerosis (hyperfiltration/collapsing)
    2. Diabetic nephropathy
    3. Other specific types
  K. Posttransplant lymphoproliferative disease
III. Idiopathic
  A. Chronic allograft nephropathy:
     Arterial intimal thickening, glomerulopathy and/or interstitial fibrosis and tubular atrophy without immunologic activity (no C4d or T cells)
IV. Recurrent primary disease
  A. Immunologic (e.g., IgA nephropathy, lupus nephritis, anti-GBM disease)
  B. Metabolic (e.g., amyloidosis, diabetes, oxalosis)
  C. Unknown (e.g., dense deposit disease, focal segmental glomerular sclerosis)

Modified from Colvin (2).

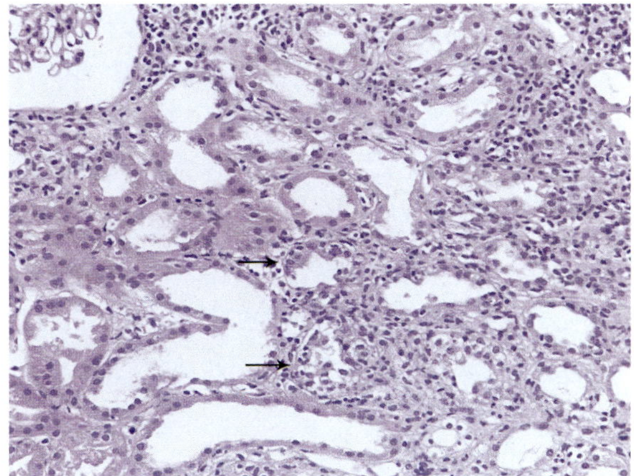

FIGURE 20.1. Acute cellular rejection (type I). A diffuse mononuclear infiltrate is present with edema and tubulitis [arrows; periodic acid-Schiff (PAS) stain].

The infiltrating mononuclear cells typically include lymphoblasts, with cytoplasmic basophilia, nucleoli, and occasional mitotic figures, indicative of increased synthetic and proliferative activity. The infiltrate consists of T cells (CD4 and CD8) macrophages and sometimes B cells.

Infiltration of mononuclear cells *under* arterial and arteriolar endothelium is the pathognomic lesion of type II acute cellular rejection ("endarteritis" or "endothelialitis") (Fig. 20.2). When lymphocytes are only on the surface of the endothelium, their significance is less certain. Lymphocytes also commonly surround vessels, a nonspecific feature, unless the cells invade the media. Endotheliitis has been reported in 48% to 54% of the renal biopsies with acute cellular rejection in three series (4–6). Some do

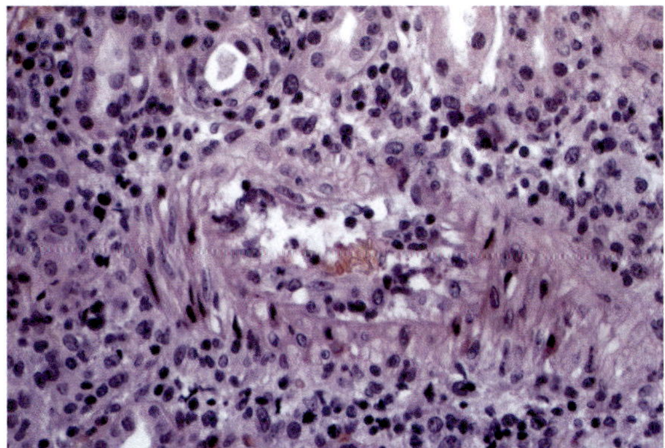

FIGURE 20.2. Acute cellular rejection with endarteritis (type II). A small artery has subendothelial infiltration of mononuclear cells 7 days after transplantation (H&E stain).

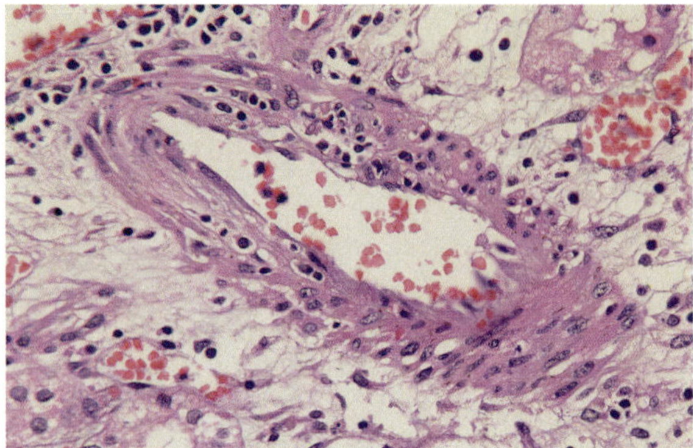

FIGURE 20.3. Acute cellular rejection, type III. Transmural inflammation of an artery is shown. The C4d stain was negative.

not find the lesion as often, which may possibly be ascribed to inadequate sampling, overdiagnosis of rejection, or timing of the biopsy with respect to antirejection therapy. These lesions are more frequent in the larger arteries (6). In our experience, about 20% of the arteries are involved, so that several arteries in the sample are almost essential for its detection (6). Rarely, the lymphocytes invade through the media, so-called transmural endarteritis (Fig. 20.3).

In most cases of acute cellular rejection, the glomeruli are spared or show minor changes, typically a few scattered mononuclear cells (T cells and monocytes) and occasionally segmental endothelial damage, termed "glomerulitis" (7–9). In a minority of cases, a severe, diffuse form of glomerular injury is evident and dominates the histologic pattern (Fig. 20.4).

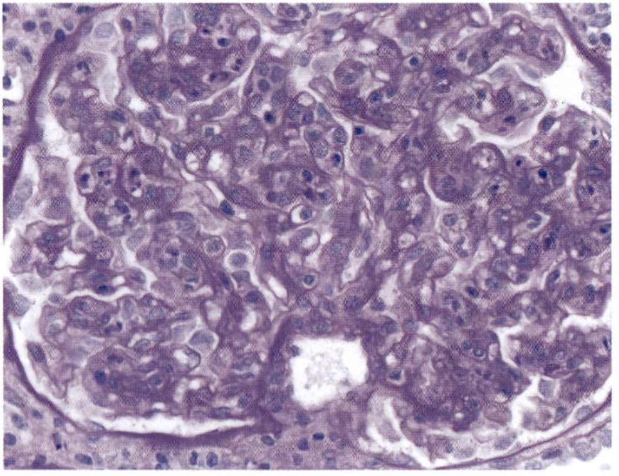

FIGURE 20.4. Acute allograft glomerulopathy. This pattern of glomerular injury can occur as a feature of cellular or humoral rejection (PAS stain).

In 1981 Richardson and his colleagues (10) drew attention to a distinctive, acute allograft glomerulopathy, characterized by hypercellularity, injury and enlargement of endothelial cells, infiltration of glomeruli by mononuclear cells, and by webs of periodic acid-Schiff (PAS)-positive material. The glomeruli contain numerous $CD3^+$ and $CD8^+$ T cells and monocytes (9,11). This severe form of glomerulopathy has been observed in 4% to 7% of biopsies taken for allograft dysfunction, typically 1 to 4 months after transplantation (10,12–14). Acute allograft glomerulopathy is believed to be an unusual variant of cellular rejection, sometimes promoted by cytomegalovirus (CMV) infection. T cells, not antibodies, are regularly detected in glomeruli immunohistochemically (9,11), and OKT3 can reverse the lesion (15). For unknown reasons, rejection becomes focused on glomerular components; florid glomerulopathy may occur with little interstitial inflammation, although cellular endarteritis is common.

Interstitial mononuclear inflammation and tubulitis occur in a variety of diseases other than acute rejection, such as drug-induced allergic tubulo-interstitial nephritis, and therefore cannot be considered proof that rejection is present. The presence of systemic infection is another well-known cause of tubulo-interstitial nephritis and tubulitis. Tubulitis has been documented in renal transplants with dysfunction due to lymphocele (obstruction) and to pneumonia (15). Tubulitis is often present in atrophic tubules from any cause and does not indicate acute rejection. Posttreatment with anti–T-cell antibodies, the inflammation diminishes in most patients and this is correlated with successful response to therapy. This type of rejection often responds to steroid pulses and rarely causes graft loss (6,16–19).

Cellular arteritis must not be confused with necrotizing arteritis, characteristic of humoral rejection (type III). Rarely, transmural cellular inflammation causes frank medial necrosis, but this complication of cellular arteritis can be distinguished from necrotizing arteritis by the heavy mononuclear infiltrate. Regrettably, many still do not distinguish these lesions, regarding all "vascular rejection" as predominately humoral. Cellular arteritis has a much better rate of reversal than necrotizing arteritis (61% vs. 29% 1-year graft survival) (20), which alone justifies their separation.

Immunofluorescence Microscopy

Immunofluorescence microscopy shows little, if any, immunoglobulin deposition, but interstitial fibrin is typically present (21). Fibrin and scant immunoglobulin and C3 deposits may also be found in glomeruli. C4d in peritubular capillaries is a marker of humoral rejection (see below).

Electron Microscopy

Electron microscopy is generally not used for the diagnosis of acute rejection. Studies have shown endothelial injury in peritubular and glomerular capillaries, invasion of lymphocytes into tubules. No immune deposits are detectable. Cases with acute allograft glomerulopathy show markedly reactive endothelial cells, with mononuclear cells in capillaries and often platelet/fibrin aggregates.

Classification of Acute Cellular Rejection (Table 20.2)

The most widely used classification system is the Banff working schema, which is now congruent with the Collaborative Clinical Trials in Transplantation (CCTT) categories (17,22). The Banff system scores each element (infiltrate, tubulitis, arteritis, glomerulitis) on a 0 to 3 scale (1, mild; 2, moderate; 3, severe) as the basis for grading. The Banff system promoted standardization of definitions; however, the interobserver reproducibility for component grading of the Banff system is disappointing, with kappa values of <0.4 (in the poor range) (23). The scoring for tubulitis and arteritis was improved by scoring photographs, indicating that finding the relevant lesion on the slide was a limiting factor; scoring of the percent infiltrate or glomerulitis was not improved by scoring a photograph, suggesting intrinsic problems in the definitions or methodology. The major remaining issues for the future are to define more markers for treatable rejection in the suspicious category and incorporate glomerular lesions in the classification.

Pathogenesis

Type I and II cellular rejection are mediated by T cells rather than antibodies, since they both occur in the absence of circulating antibody or evidence of complement fixation in the graft. In animals cellular endarteritis occurs

TABLE 20.2 Banff classification of acute rejection (39)[1]

Acute cellular rejection (T-cell mediated)	Acute humoral rejection[2] (antibody mediated)
Suspicious/borderline[3]	
Type I: tubulointerstitial	Type I: acute tubular injury
Type II: endarteritis	Type II: capillary inflammation
Type III: arterial transmural inflammation (or fibrinoid necrosis)[4]	Type III: fibrinoid arterial necrosis (or transmural inflammation)[5]

[1] Cellular and humoral acute rejection commonly occur together, and both can be diagnosed if the criteria for each are met.

[2] Requires demonstration of C4d deposition in peritubular capillaries or immunoglobulin and complement in arterial walls.

[3] Includes infiltrates of 10–25% with tubulitis. The CCTT system considers these acute cellular rejection (17).

[4] Most of the cases with fibrinoid necrosis of arteries are due to humoral rejection, but this category remains in the current Banff system.

[5] Most of the cases with transmural inflammation are expected to be cell mediated, although this has not been formally studied.

in the absence of humoral antibody (e.g., B-cell–deficient mice) (24). In humans, rejection with vascular infiltrates can usually be reversed with OKT3 (5,6,25). Both $CD8^+$ and $CD4^+$ cells invade the intima in early grafts, but later $CD8^+$ cells predominate (9,26). Arterial endothelium shows increased human leukocyte antigen DR (HLA-DR), intercellular adhesion molecule 1 (ICAM-1), and vascular cell adhesion molecule 1 (VCAM-1) in acute rejection (26,27) and the tubular epithelium shows increased HLA-DR (28). Increased expression of major histocompatibility complex (MHC) antigen and adhesion molecules are believed to be a response to cytokines. Among the most specific and sensitive measures of rejection by polymerase chain reaction (PCR) are messenger RNAs (mRNAs) for granzyme B, perforin, Fas and Fas ligand, and granulysin (29–31). A combination of two of the three markers is highly predictive of acute rejection, more so than the cytokines. This argues that the cytolytic pathway is more active than the cytokine delayed hypersensitivity mechanisms, but that applies only to the time of the biopsy, which is relatively late in the inflammatory process.

Clinicopathologic Correlations

In all large studies, endarteritis has a worse prognosis than tubulointerstitial rejection (6,16–18,32). Cases with endarteritis are less responsive to steroid pulses, but do respond to OKT3 or anti-thymocyte globulin (ATG), and have a decreased 1-year survival (6). Later development of intimal fibrosis is correlated prior type II rejection (33). Eikmans and colleagues (34) have shown that transforming growth factor-β (TGF-β) mRNA in biopsies is associated with better outcome, perhaps related to its expression in T-regulatory cells (34).

Acute Humoral Rejection (AHR), or Acute Antibody-Mediated Rejection

Clinical

The clinical features of AHR consist of severe and acute (days) graft dysfunction that is not responsive to steroids or usually antilymphocytes antibodies and with a higher rate of graft loss than cellular rejection. It can arise any time after transplant. The risk factors for AHR include elevated panel reactive antibody (PRA), prior transplant, and historically positive cross-match, all associated with prior sensitization (35–38). Patients who reduce immunosuppression late after transplant, either due to noncompliance or nonabsorption, can manifest AHR.

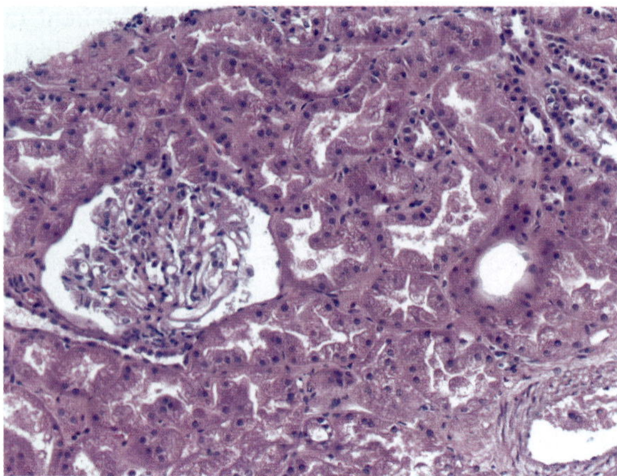

FIGURE 20.5. Humoral rejection, type I. Acute tubular injury is evident, without neutrophils in capillaries. The C4d stain was positive.

Pathologic Findings

Light Microscopy

Three forms of AHR have been recognized (Figs. 20.5 to 20.7) (19,39): (1) acute tubular injury with little inflammation, (2) peritubular and glomerular capillary inflammation with neutrophils, and (3) necrosis of arteries. Acute humoral rejection can be missed in routine sections. In one series, a component of AHR would not have been recognized in 25% of cases

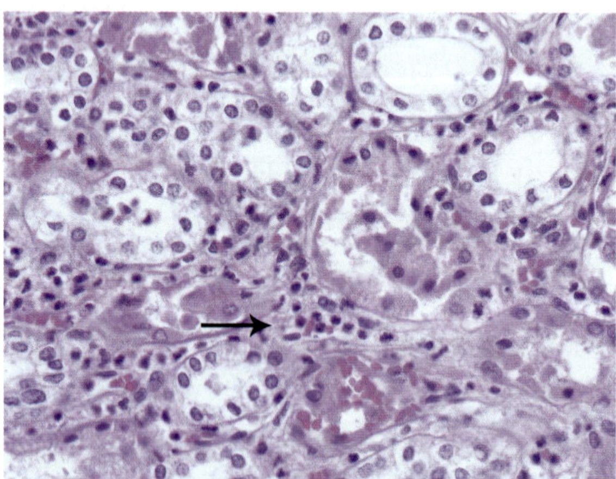

FIGURE 20.6. Humoral rejection, type II. Neutrophils are in peritubular capillaries and glomeruli; interstitial hemorrhage is present. Anti–donor class II antibodies were demonstrable (H&E stain).

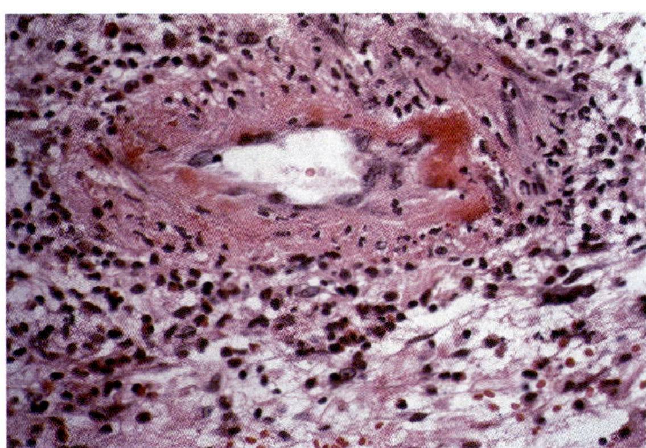

FIGURE 20.7. Acute humoral rejection with fibrinoid necrosis (type III). A small artery has fibrin and necrosis in the media with a scanty infiltrate (H&E stain).

without the C4d stain: 15% showed only ACR and 10% only acute tubular injury (19). The 10% acute tubular injury biopsies comprised of two donor specific antibodies (DSA$^+$) patients with widespread C4d staining of peritubular capillaries (PTCs) that showed predominantly acute tubular injury on initial biopsy (Fig. 20.5). Later biopsies performed in one of these showed typical AHR with abundant neutrophils in PTCs and glomeruli as well as fibrinoid necrosis. Most cases have neutrophils in PTCs (Fig. 20.6). This feature is useful, but not highly sensitive or specific (19). The histologic features in the Regele et al (36) series were similarly misleading: 32% of those with C4d did not meet the Banff criteria for rejection, accounting for about 75% of the patients with AHR. In some cases arterial and arteriolar thrombosis and glomerular thrombosis and necrosis predominate similarly to thrombotic microangiopathy (37–39). These lesions must be distinguished from the hemolytic-uremic syndrome of calcineurin inhibitor toxicity, which can also have thrombi in arterioles and glomeruli, but does not affect the peritubular capillaries (or have C4d). A minority of cases have fibrinoid necrosis, in which the arterial media shows myocyte necrosis, fragmentation of elastica, and accumulation of brightly eosinophilic material called "fibrinoid" and little mononuclear infiltrate in the intima or adventitia (Fig. 20.7). A scant infiltrate of neutrophils and eosinophils and thrombosis may be present.

Immunofluorescence Microscopy

Detection of C4d has proved to be useful in the detection of humoral rejection (Fig. 20.8). After antibody binds to antigen, C4 is proteolytically cleaved by activated C1 into C4a and C4b. The cleavage of C4 exposes the reactive and short-lived thiol group in C4b that binds covalently to nearby molecules containing amino or hydroxyl groups, such as proteins and carbohydrates (40,41). Bound C4b is proteolytically inactivated into

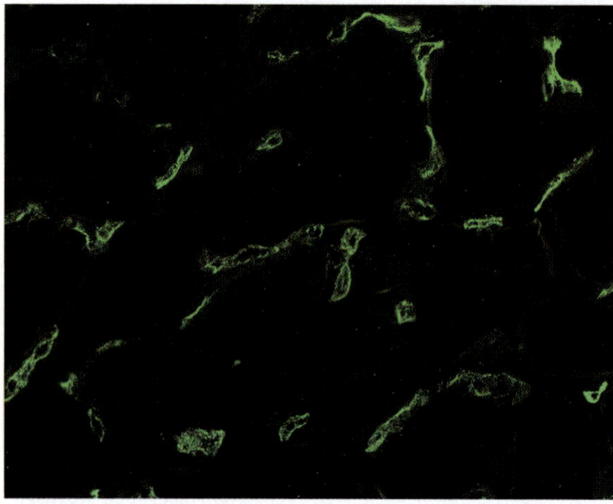

FIGURE 20.8. Acute humoral rejection. C4d is present in peritubular capillaries (immunofluorescence on frozen section; monoclonal antibody to C4d).

C4d, a 44.5-kd peptide, which contains the thioester site and remains covalently bound at the same site. Thus, if C4d is bound to a structural protein, it is potentially a durable marker of local complement activation by the classical pathway. C4d can disappear as soon as 8 days (28), and after 60 days is usually negative (unless chronic humoral rejection develops) (19). Cases with fibrinoid necrosis of arteries typically contain immunoglobulin (Ig; usually IgG and IgM), C3, and fibrin in the arterial walls. The criteria for acute humoral rejection proposed by Mauiyyedi et al (19) and accepted with minor modification by the Banff conference are given in Table 20.3 (39):

Pathogenesis

Donor specific anti-HLA antibodies are detected in 90% of C4d$^+$ acute rejection cases compared with 2% in C4d$^-$ acute rejection cases ($p < 0.001$) (19). We have speculated that the DSA-negative cases are due to adsorption in the graft or to non-HLA specificities. Circulating pretransplant and post-transplant DSA can be identified by T- and B-cell cytotoxicity assays or flow cytometry, as well as panel reactive analysis (PRA) and flow-PRA

TABLE 20.3. Criteria for acute humoral rejection (AHR)[1]

1. Widespread, linear C4d$^+$ staining of peritubular capillaries
2. Evidence for acute renal injury consisting of at least one of the following:
   a. Acute tubular injury
   b. Neutrophils in peritubular or glomerular capillaries
   c. Fibrinoid necrosis of arteries
3. Circulating anti–donor-specific antibodies

[1] If only two of the three major criteria are established (for example, when no human leukocyte antigen cross-match is available or when C4d staining is not done), the diagnosis should be considered suspicious for AHR.

(35, 37). Although most patients are negative pretransplant for DSA, presensitization accounts for some of the C4d$^+$ cases (18,28,42). Repeat testing with the most sensitive techniques sometimes reveals an occult DSA. The circulating antibodies in AHR are usually to donor HLA class I antigens (43), although about 30% show only reactivity to class II MHC antigens (35,44,45), or to non-MHC molecules on endothelium (46–48). C4d will presumably be deposited in cases of AHR due to non-HLA antibodies, and therefore has potential value as an antigen-independent test for humoral rejection.

Clinicopathologic Correlations

A substantial fraction (about 25–50%) of acute renal allograft rejection episodes have a component of AHR as judged by C4d deposition in PTC (32). In one series 30% of patients with biopsy-confirmed acute rejection had a humoral rejection component as judged by widespread C4d staining of the PTC, representing 9% of renal transplant patients overall (32). The overall graft loss at 1 year after AHR is considerably worse than after ACR. In a large, well-analyzed study, the presence of C4d strikingly and adversely impacted the outcome of either type 1 (tubulitis) or type 2 (endarteritis) acute rejection (18).

Hyperacute Rejection

Hyperacute rejection occurs when the recipient is presensitized to donor antigens expressed by the endothelium, usually HLA or ABO antigens. Graft dysfunction occurs within minutes to hours of reperfusion, and the grafts generally never function. The pathology is similar to that described for acute humoral rejection, including neutrophils in capillaries, thrombi, and hemorrhage (Fig. 20.9). C4d is generally demonstrable in peritubular capillaries. With ABO incompatibility, IgM is often detectable (Fig. 20.10).

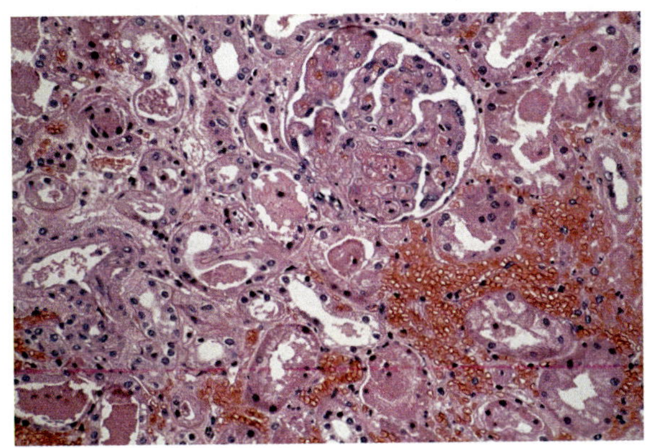

FIGURE 20.9. Hyperacute rejection. The cortex shows diffuse hemorrhage and neutrophils in peritubular capillaries with prominent glomerular thrombi 1 day after transplantation (H&E stain).

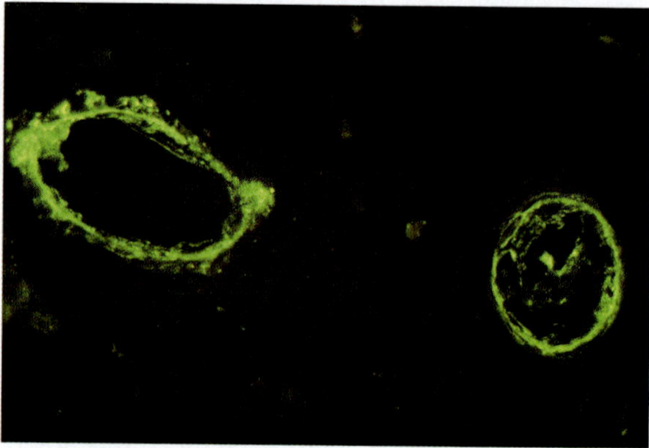

FIGURE 20.10. Hyperacute rejection due to ABO incompatibility. Immunofluorescence stain shows immunoglobulin M (IgM) in arterial walls.

Chronic Rejection

Introduction/Clinical Setting

The rate of long-term graft loss changed little over the last decade, despite dramatic improvements in short-term graft survival. The clinical features of late graft dysfunction are a slowly rising creatinine, often accompanied by severe proteinuria and hypertension. Graft function may be lost gradually over a period of months to years, with or without episodes of acute rejection. The rate of graft loss is steady after the initial 3 to 6 months, with a half-life of 7.2 years for cadaver donor grafts, 10.8 years for parent-to-child grafts, and 26.9 years for grafts from HLA-identical siblings (49). Most late graft loss, other than patient death, has been attributed to chronic allograft nephropathy (CAN). Despite (or perhaps because of) the ambiguous use of the term, CAN publications have increased exponentially since 1993 (50).

Chronic allograft nephropathy entered primetime in 1993 as a category in the Banff working classification that was to include "at least four entities that at present cannot always be distinguished by biopsy (chronic rejection, chronic cyclosporine toxicity, hypertensive vascular disease, and chronic infection and/or reflux)" (50). The rationale was that "because it is often impossible to define the precise cause or causes of chronic allograft damage, the term 'chronic/sclerosing allograft nephropathy' is preferable to 'chronic rejection,' which implies allogeneic mechanisms of injury, *unless* there are specific features to incriminate such a rejection process" (emphasis added) (22). A rejection process was suggested according to the Banff classification by intimal fibrosis with inflammatory cells and duplication of the glomerular basement membrane (GBM) (22). Chronic allograft nephropathy was *not* intended to replace specific diagnostic categories, *if* these entities could be identified.

Unfortunately, CAN is often misused as a generic term for chronic renal allograft dysfunction and fibrosis, or as a synonym for "chronic rejection." If indiscriminately applied to all causes of renal allograft dysfunction with fibrosis, the term inhibits accurate diagnosis and appropriate therapy and therefore has little value, other than to hide our ignorance. In my view and according to the original Banff conception, CAN should be restricted to the minority of biopsies that are truly nonspecific in their pathology [i.e., CAN, not otherwise specified (CANNOS)] (51). When an alloimmune basis can be identified in the pathogenesis, the term *chronic rejection* is most appropriate.

Pathologic Findings

Light Microscopy

The arterial lesion is the cardinal feature of chronic rejection (Fig. 20.11) (52). The arteries show pronounced fibrous intimal thickening with myointimal cells, collagen fibrils, focal calcification, a variable infiltrate of T cells (often subendothelial), and lipid-filled, foamy macrophages disposed characteristically against the external elastica, which is duplicated and disrupted. The adventitia also often has an infiltrate of mononuclear cells, sometimes invading and destroying the outer media. Marked duplication of the internal elastica, a normal or thickened media, and relative sparing of the larger arteries (arcuate and larger) are more typical of hypertension (53). The arterioles are relatively spared in chronic rejection, compared with chronic cyclosporin A (CsA) toxicity, thrombotic microangiopathy/

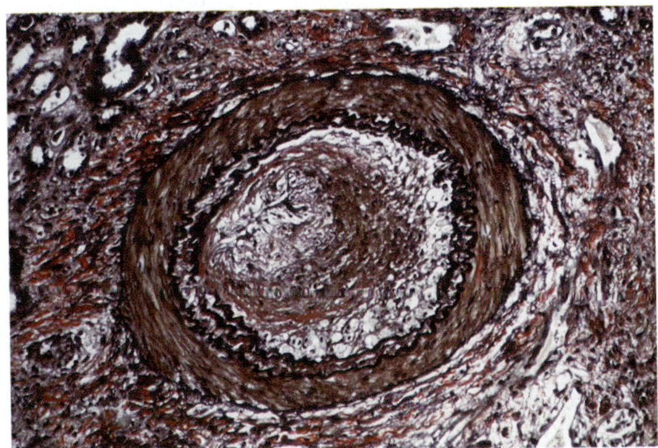

FIGURE 20.11. Chronic allograft arteriopathy. Expansion of the intima with foam cells and scattered infiltrating mononuclear cells are shown in a nephrectomy 2 years after transplantation (elastin stain).

hemolytic uremic syndrome, and systemic sclerosis. These processes do not cause a mononuclear infiltrate in the vessels. However, the healing phase of hemolytic uremic syndrome and systemic sclerosis may leave intimal fibrosis that resembles chronic rejection.

The glomerular features are not specific for chronic graft rejection, but are typical. The glomeruli have an increase in mesangial cells and matrix and thickening and duplication of the GBM, with various degrees of scarring and adhesions (Fig. 20.12). This lesion has been shown to derive from acute allograft glomerulopathy in a few cases (10,14). Extensive crescents, diffuse granular or linear deposits of IgG, or subepithelial deposits are unusual and suggest recurrent or de novo glomerulonephritis.

Immunofluorescence Microscopy

Immunofluorescence shows segmental or granular deposits of immunoglobulin (typically IgM and IgG, rarely IgA), C3, and sometimes fibrin in the capillary wall and in the mesangium. C4d deposition in peritubular capillaries is found in about 50% of patients with CAG or CAA. Glomerular C4d deposition is often detectable in paraffin sections.

Electron Microscopy

Electron microscopy shows foot process effacement and focal mesangial cell interposition, and mesangiolysis may be present (54). Endothelial cell "dedifferentiation" is often evident, as manifested by a loss of the normal fenestrations (55,56). Loss of this normal differentiated structure of glomerular endothelial cells should markedly restrict bulk water flow through the capillary wall and decrease filtration. The other diseases with similar

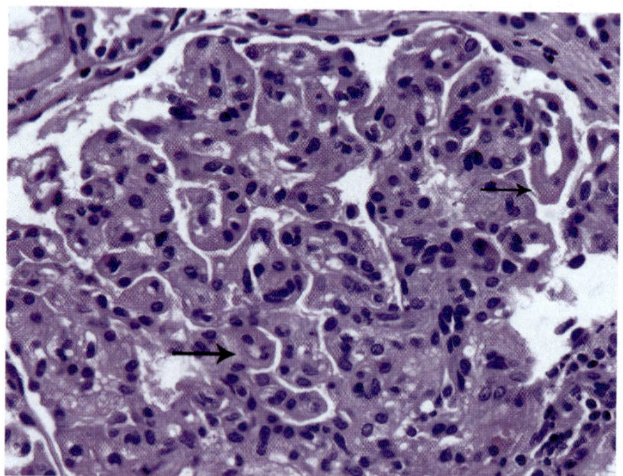

Figure 20.12. Chronic allograft glomerulopathy. Mesangial hypercellularity and duplication of the glomerular basement membrane (GBM) are prominent (arrow; PAS stain).

light and electron microscopic glomerular features also are characterized by endothelial injury (thrombotic microangiopathy, scleroderma, and eclampsia). A chronic lesion in the peritubular capillaries has been observed consisting of splitting and multilayered duplication of the basement membrane, analogous to and correlated with the chronic glomerular changes (57). Thus, the common theme in chronic rejection is endothelial damage at the level of the arteries, glomeruli, and peritubular capillaries.

Pathogenesis

Previous studies with classic HLA techniques had reported that de novo antibodies to graft HLA class I and II antigens were risk factors for chronic transplant arteriopathy (58,59) and predicted graft loss (60,61). New evidence has connected circulating DSA specifically with complement fixation and pathology in the graft. We reported that biopsies in the majority of chronic rejection (CAG or CAA) in humans have a detectable humoral component (62) as judged by C4d deposition and circulating DSA. This suggests that antibodies that fix complement at the level of the PTCs mediate a major subset of chronic rejection. Others have confirmed and extended these observations. Regele et al (36) showed that 73 of 213 (34%) of graft biopsies taken >12 months posttransplant had C4d in PTC. C4d was correlated with CAG and lamination of the PTC basement membrane: 66% of the cases with CAG had C4d (similar to the 61% in our study). Most importantly, C4d was found to *precede and predict* the later development of CAG, arguing that it is related to the pathogenesis and not just an incidental finding. The prevalence of humoral rejection may vary with the immunosuppressive protocol, but no current therapy prevents humoral rejection; cases have occurred with cyclosporine, azathioprine, mycophenolate, CAMPATH1, FTY720, and tacrolimus (37,62–65). Overall, among five reports comprising 353 patients, 51% of those with CAG/CAA (n = 136) had C4d deposition in PTC vs. 10% of grafts without evidence of chronic rejection (n = 217) (62,66–69). Finally, microarray analysis of gene expression in human renal allograft biopsies revealed that B-cell infiltrate predicts increased risk of graft loss due to rejection (70).

A consensus meeting at the National Institutes of Health (NIH) established draft criteria for chronic humoral rejection (CHR) and four theoretical stages in the development of CHR (71). According to this schema, the first evidence of humoral response is the new appearance of DSA (stage I). In some cases this rapidly progresses to AHR. In other cases, for unknown reasons, DSA does not elicit an immediate acute rejection. The next stage (II) shows evidence of antibody interacting with graft endothelium in the form of C4d deposition in PTC, but without graft damage, as judged by normal histology and function. The ensuing stages proceed to pathologic injury (III) and finally clinical evidence of graft dysfunction (azotemia, proteinuria). This sequence has been observed in non-human primates (72). Other possibilities can be considered. DSA may not be detectable in the circulation immediately, due to adsorption by the graft. C4d may appear in the graft before antibody "overflows" to the circulation. Regression may occur if antibody ceases to be produced or is intermittent. C4d may not necessarily lead to pathologic injury (e.g., accommodation).

Differential Diagnosis

The glomerular features are not specific for chronic graft rejection, but are typical. The most distinctive features in my opinion are the loss of endothelial fenestrations and duplication of the GBM. The other diseases with similar light and electron microscopic glomerular features also are characterized by endothelial injury (thrombotic microangiopathy, scleroderma, eclampsia). If immune complex deposits are more than occasionally found, or if in a subepithelial location, recurrent or de novo glomerulonephritis should be suspected. The features that favor chronic rejection over chronic CsA toxicity are duplication of the GBM and marked intimal fibrosis of the small arteries. Atypical, monomorphic infiltrates particularly with necrosis, are highly suspicious of post-transplant lymphoproliferative disease (PTLD). Peripheral hyalinosis replacing smooth muscle cells in the arterioles favors CsA toxicity.

References

1. Pascual M, Vallhonrat H, Cosimi AB, et al. The clinical usefulness of the renal allograft biopsy in the cyclosporine era: a prospective study. Transplantation 67:737–741, 1999.
2. Colvin RB. Renal transplant pathology. In: Jennette JC, Olson JL, Schwartz MM, Silva FG, eds. Heptinstall's Pathology of the Kidney, Philadelphia: Lippincott-Raven, 1998:1409–1540.
3. Colvin RB. Pathology of the renal allograft. In: Renal Biopsy in Medical Diseases of the Kidneys. New York: Columbia University Medical Center, 2004.
4. Sibley RK, Rynasiewicz J, Ferguson RM, et al. Morphology of cyclosporine nephrotoxicity and acute rejection in patients immunosuppressed with cyclosporine and prednisone. Surgery 94:225–234, 1983.
5. Schroeder TJ, Weiss MA, Smith RD, Stephens GW, First MR. The efficacy of OKT3 in vascular rejection. Transplantation 51:312–315, 1991.
6. Nickeleit V, Vamvakas EC, Pascual M, Poletti BJ, Colvin RB. The prognostic significance of specific arterial lesions in acute renal allograft rejection. J Am Soc Nephrol 9:1301–1308, 1998.
7. Bishop GA, Hall BM, Duggin GG, Horvath JS, Sheil AG, Tiller DJ. Immunopathology of renal allograft rejection analyzed with monoclonal antibodies to mononuclear cell markers. Kidney Int 29:708–717, 1986.
8. Harry TR, Coles GA, Davies M, Bryant D, Williams GT, Griffin PJ. The significance of monocytes in glomeruli of human renal transplants. Transplantation 37:70–73, 1984.

9. Tuazon TV, Schneeberger EE, Bhan AK, et al. Mononuclear cells in acute allograft glomerulopathy. Am J Pathol 129:119–132, 1987.
10. Richardson WP, Colvin RB, Cheeseman SH, et al. Glomerulopathy associated with cytomegalovirus viremia in renal allografts. N Engl J Med 305:57–63, 1981.
11. Hiki Y, Leong AY, Mathew TH, Seymour AE, Pascoe V, Woodroofe AJ. Typing of intraglomerular mononuclear cells associated with transplant glomerular rejection. Clin Nephrol 26:244–249, 1986.
12. Axelsen RA, Seymour AE, Mathew TH, Canny A, Pascoe V. Glomerular transplant rejection: a distinctive pattern of early graft damage. Clin Nephrol 23:1–11, 1985.
13. Herrera GA, Alexander RW, Cooley CF, et al. Cytomegalovirus glomerulopathy: a controversial lesion. Kidney Int 29:725–733, 1986.
14. Maryniak R, First RM, Weiss MA. Transplant glomerulopathy: evolution of morphologically distinct changes. Kidney Int 27:799–806, 1985.
15. Hibberd AD, Nanra RS, White KH, Trevillian PR. Reversal of acute glomerular renal allograft rejection: a possible effect of OKT3. Transplant Int 4:246–248, 1991.
16. Bates WD, Davies DR, Welsh K, Gray DW, Fuggle SV, Morris PJ. An evaluation of the Banff classification of early renal allograft biopsies and correlation with outcome. Nephrol Dialysis Transplant 14:2364–2369, 1999.
17. Colvin RB, Cohen AH, Saiontz C, et al. Evaluation of pathologic criteria for acute renal allograft rejection: reproducibility, sensitivity, and clinical correlation. J Am Soc Nephrol 8:1930–1941, 1997.
18. Herzenberg AM, Gill JS, Djurdjev O, Magil AB. C4d deposition in acute rejection: an independent long-term prognostic factor. J Am Soc Nephrol 13:234–241, 2002.
19. Mauiyyedi S, Crespo M, Collins AB, et al. Acute humoral rejection in kidney transplantation: II. Morphology, immunopathology, and pathologic classification. J Am Soc Nephrol 13:779–787, 2002.
20. Matas AJ, Sibley R, Mauer M, Sutherland DE, Simmons RL, Najarian JS. The value of needle renal allograft biopsy. I. A retrospective study of biopsies performed during putative rejection episodes. Ann Surg 197:226–237, 1983.
21. Gould VE, Martinez LV, Virtanen I, Sahlin KM, Schwartz MM. Differential distribution of tenascin and cellular fibronectins in acute and chronic renal allograft rejection. Lab Invest 67:71–79, 1992.
22. Racusen LC, Solez K, Colvin RB, et al. The Banff 97 working classification of renal allograft pathology. Kidney Int 55:713–723, 1999.
23. Furness PN, Taub N, Assmann KJ, et al. International variation in histologic grading is large, and persistent feedback does not improve reproducibility. Am J Surg Pathol 27:805–810, 2003.
24. Russell PS, Chase CM, Colvin RB. Contributions of cellular and humoral immunity to arteriopathic lesions in transplanted mouse hearts. Transplant Proc 29:2527–2528, 1997.
25. Visscher D, Carey J, Oh H, et al. Histologic and immunophenotypic evaluation of pretreatment renal biopsies in OKT3-treated allograft rejections. Transplantation 51:1023–1028, 1991.
26. Alpers CE, Hudkins KL, Davis CL, et al. Expression of vascular cell adhesion molecule-1 in kidney allograft rejection. Kidney Int 44:805–816, 1993.

27. Brockmeyer C, Ulbrecht M, Schendel DJ, et al. Distribution of cell adhesion molecules (ICAM-1, VCAM-1, ELAM-1) in renal tissue during allograft rejection. Transplantation 55:610–615, 1993.
28. Nickeleit V, Zeiler M, Gudat F, Thiel G, Mihatsch MJ. Detection of the complement degradation product C4d in renal allografts: diagnostic and therapeutic implications. J Am Soc Nephrol 13:242–251, 2002.
29. Strehlau J, Pavlakis M, Lipman M, et al. Quantitative detection of immune activation transcripts as a diagnostic tool in kidney transplantation. Proc Natl Acad Sci USA 94:695–700, 1997.
30. Sharma VK, Bologa RM, Li B, et al. Molecular executors of cell death—differential intrarenal expression of Fas ligand, Fas, granzyme B, and perforin during acute and/or chronic rejection of human renal allografts. Transplantation 62:1860–1866, 1996.
31. Sarwal MM, Jani A, Chang S, et al. Granulysin expression is a marker for acute rejection and steroid resistance in human renal transplantation. Hum Immunol 62:21–31, 2001.
32. Mauiyyedi S, Colvin RB. Humoral rejection in kidney transplantation: new concepts in diagnosis and treatment. Curr Opin Nephrol Hypertens 11:609–618, 2002.
33. Nankivell BJ, Fenton-Lee CA, Kuypers DR, et al. Effect of histological damage on long-term kidney transplant outcome. Transplantation 71:515–523, 2001.
34. Eikmans M, Sijpkens YW, Baelde HJ, de Heer E, Paul LC, Bruijn JA. High transforming growth factor-beta and extracellular matrix mRNA response in renal allografts during early acute rejection is associated with absence of chronic rejection. Transplantation 73:573–579, 2002.
35. Crespo M, Pascual M, Tolkoff-Rubin N, et al. Acute humoral rejection in renal allograft recipients: I. Incidence, serology and clinical characteristics. Transplantation 71:652–658, 2001.
36. Regele H, Exner M, Watschinger B, et al. Endothelial C4d deposition is associated with inferior kidney allograft outcome independently of cellular rejection. Nephrol Dial Transplant 16:2058–2066, 2001.
37. Bohmig GA, Exner M, Habicht A, et al. Capillary C4d deposition in kidney allografts: a specific marker of alloantibody-dependent graft injury. J Am Soc Nephrol 13:1091–1099, 2002.
38. Lederer SR, Kluth-Pepper B, Schneeberger H, Albert E, Land W, Feucht HE. Impact of humoral alloreactivity early after transplantation on the long-term survival of renal allografts. Kidney Int 59:334–341, 2001.
39. Racusen LC, Colvin RB, Solez K, et al. Antibody-mediated rejection criteria—an addition to the Banff 97 classification of renal allograft rejection. Am J Transplant 3:708–714, 2003.
40. Campbell RD, Gagnon J, Porter RR. Amino acid sequence around the thiol and reactive acyl groups of human complement component C4. Biochem J 199:359–370, 1981.
41. Harrison RA, Thomas ML, Tack BF. Sequence determination of the thiolester site of the fourth component of human complement. Proc Natl Acad Sci USA 78:7388–7392, 1981.
42. Feucht HE, Schneeberger H, Hillebrand G, et al. Capillary deposition of C4d complement fragment and early renal graft loss. Kidney Int 43:1333–1338, 1993.

43. Halloran PF, Schlaut J, Solez K, Srinivasa NS. The significance of the anti-class I antibody response. II. Clinical and pathologic features of renal transplants with anti-class I-like antibody. Transplantation 53:550–555, 1992.
44. Scornik JC, LeFor WM, Cicciarelli JC, et al. Hyperacute and acute kidney graft rejection due to antibodies against B cells. Transplantation 54:61–64, 1992.
45. Russ GR, Nicholls C, Sheldon A, Hay J. Positive B cell crossmatch and glomerular rejection in renal transplant recipients. Transplant Proc 19:2837–2839, 1987.
46. Kooijmans-Coutinho MF, Hermans J, Schrama E, et al. Interstitial rejection, vascular rejection, and diffuse thrombosis of renal allografts. Predisposing factors, histology, immunohistochemistry, and relation to outcome. Transplantation 61:1338–1344, 1996.
47. Moraes JR, Stastny P. A new antigen system expressed in human endothelial cells. J Clin Invest 60:449–454, 1971.
48. Zwirner NW, Dole K, Stastny P. Differential surface expression of MICA by endothelial cells, fibroblasts, keratinocytes, and monocytes. Hum Immunol 60:323–330, 1999.
49. Terasaki P, Cecka JM. Worldwide transplant center directory. In: Terasaki P, Cecka JM, eds. Clinical Transplants 1991. Los Angeles: UCLA Tissue Typing Laboratory, 1992:579.
50. Solez K, Axelsen RA, Benediktsson H, et al. International standardization of criteria for the histologic diagnosis of renal allograft rejection: the Banff working classification of kidney transplant pathology. Kidney Int 44:411–422, 1993.
51. Colvin RB. Chronic allograft nephropathy. N Engl J Med 349:2288–2290, 2003.
52. Sibley RK. Morphologic features of chronic rejection in kidney and less commonly transplanted organs. Clin Transplant 8:293–298, 1994.
53. Porter KA. Renal transplantation. In: Heptinstall RH, ed. The Pathology of the Kidney, Boston: Little, Brown, 1990:1799–1933.
54. Hsu HC, Suzuki Y, Churg J, Grishman E. Ultrastructure of transplant glomerulopathy. Histopathology 4:351–367, 1980.
55. Colvin RB. Pathology of renal allografts. In: Colvin RB, Bhan AK, McCluskey RT, eds. Diagnostic Immunopathology, New York: Raven Press, 1995:329–366.
56. Cosio FG, Roche Z, Agarwal A, Falkenhain ME, Sedmak DD, Ferguson RM. Prevalence of hepatitis C in patients with idiopathic glomerulonephritis in native and transplant kidneys. Am J Kidney Dis 28:752–758, 1996.
57. Mazzucco G, Motta M, Segoloni G, Monga G. Intertubular capillary changes in the cortex and medulla of transplanted kidneys and their relationship with transplant glomerulopathy: an ultrastructural study of 12 transplantectomies. Ultrastruct Pathol 18:533–537, 1994.
58. Jeannet M, Pinn VW, Flax MH, Winn HJ, Russell PS. Humoral antibodies in renal allotransplantation in man. N Engl J Med 282:111–117, 1970.
59. Davenport A, Younie ME, Parsons JE, Klouda PT. Development of cytotoxic antibodies following renal allograft transplantation is associated with reduced graft survival due to chronic vascular rejection. Nephrol Dialysis Transplant 9:1315–1319, 1994.

60. Piazza A, Poggi E, Borrelli L, et al. Impact of donor-specific antibodies on chronic rejection occurrence and graft loss in renal transplantation: posttransplant analysis using flow cytometric techniques. Transplantation 71:1106–1112, 2001.
61. Pelletier RP, Hennessy PK, Adams PW, VanBuskirk AM, Ferguson RM, Orosz CG. Clinical significance of MHC-reactive alloantibodies that develop after kidney or kidney-pancreas transplantation. Am J Transplant 2:134–141, 2002.
62. Mauiyyedi S, Pelle PD, Saidman S, et al. Chronic humoral rejection: identification of antibody-mediated chronic renal allograft rejection by C4d deposits in peritubular capillaries. J Am Soc Nephrol 12:574–582, 2001.
63. Magil AB, Tinckam K. Monocytes and peritubular capillary C4d deposition in acute renal allograft rejection. Kidney Int 63:1888–1893, 2003.
64. Knechtle SJ, Pirsch JD, Fechner JJ, et al. Campath-1H induction plus rapamycin monotherapy for renal transplantation: results of a pilot study. Am J Transplant 3:722–730, 2003.
65. Nadasdy T, Nadasdy GM, Proca D, Yearsley K, Ferguson RM. High incidence of C4d positive humoral rejection in renal transplant patients treated with FTY720. Modern Pathology 17:290A, 2004.
66. Regele H, Bohmig GA, Habicht A, et al. Capillary deposition of complement split product C4d in renal allografts is associated with basement membrane injury in peritubular and glomerular capillaries: a contribution of humoral immunity to chronic allograft rejection. J Am Soc Nephrol 13:2371–2380, 2002.
67. Mroz A, Durlik M, Cieciura T, et al. C4d complement split product expression in chronic rejection of renal allograft. Transplant Proc 35:2190–2192, 2003.
68. Vongwiwatana A, Gourishankar S, Campbell PM, Solez K, Halloran PF. Peritubular capillary changes and C4d deposits are associated with transplant glomerulopathy but not IgA nephropathy. Am J Transplant 4:124–129, 2004.
69. Sijpkens YW, Joosten SA, Wong MC, et al. Immunologic risk factors and glomerular C4d deposits in chronic transplant glomerulopathy. Kidney Int 65:2409–2418, 2004.
70. Sarwal M, Chua MS, Kambham N, et al. Molecular heterogeneity in acute renal allograft rejection identified by DNA microarray profiling. N Engl J Med 349:125–138, 2003.
71. Takemoto SK, Zeevi A, Feng S, et al. National conference to assess antibody-mediated rejection in solid organ transplantation. Am J Transplant 4:1033–1041, 2004.
72. Smith RN, Kawai T, Boskovic S, Cardarelli F, Saidman S, Dorer D, Nadazdin O, Sachs DH, Cosimi AB, Colvin RB. Chronic antibody mediated rejection of renal allografts: pathological, serological and immunologic features in a nonhuman primate. Am J Transplant, in press.

21
Calcineurin Inhibitor Toxicity, Polyoma Virus, and Recurrent Disease

Robert B. Colvin

Calcineurin Inhibitor Toxicity (CIT)

Introduction/Clinical Setting

Cyclosporin A (CsA) has greatly improved graft survival since its introduction in the early 1980s. Tacrolimus is used clinically as an alternative to CsA, and while the drugs are structurally unrelated, their mechanism of immunosuppression is remarkably similar. The dramatic immunosuppressive and nephrotoxic effects of CsA and tacrolimus are largely explained by their calcineurin inhibition. The pathology of CsA and tacrolimus toxicity is pathologically indistinguishable.

Pathologic Findings

There are three pathologic forms of toxicity: acute nephrotoxicity, chronic nephrotoxicity, and thrombotic microangiopathy (hemolytic-uremic syndrome). Each can also arise in native kidneys in patients on CsA or tacrolimus for other reasons.

Acute Tubulopathy

The biopsy features of acute toxicity range from no morphologic abnormality to acute tubular injury or marked tubular vacuolization and vascular smooth muscle apoptosis (Fig. 21.1). The proximal tubules show loss of brush borders and isometric clear vacuolization (defined as cells filled with uniformly sized vacuoles). The vacuoles, much smaller than the nucleus, contain clear aqueous fluid rather than lipid, and are indistinguishable from those caused by osmotic diuretics. Immunofluorescence microscopy is negative. By electron microscopy, the vacuoles are dilated endoplasmic reticulum and appear empty (1). These lesions are reversible with decreased dosage.

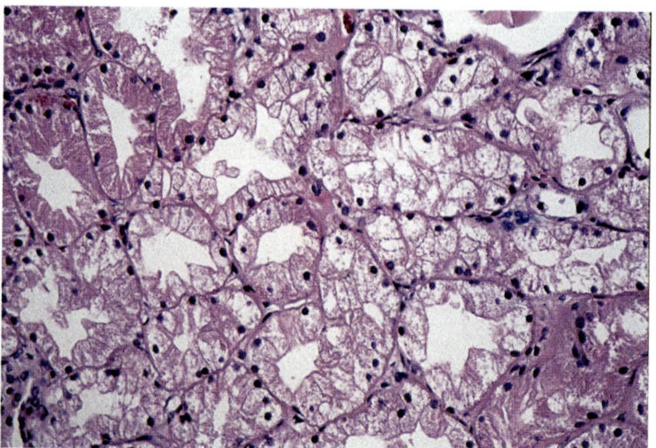

FIGURE 21.1. Acute calcineurin inhibitor toxicity, showing isometric vacuolization of proximal tubules (H&E stain).

Arteriolopathy

A spectrum of acute and chronic arteriolopathy has been described by Mihatsch, ranging from acute, focal myocyte necrosis and mucoid intimal thickening to indolent nodular hyaline deposits (Fig. 21.2) (2). The characteristic features are individual smooth muscle cell degeneration, vacuolization, necrosis, and loss. The myocytes are replaced by hyaline deposits,

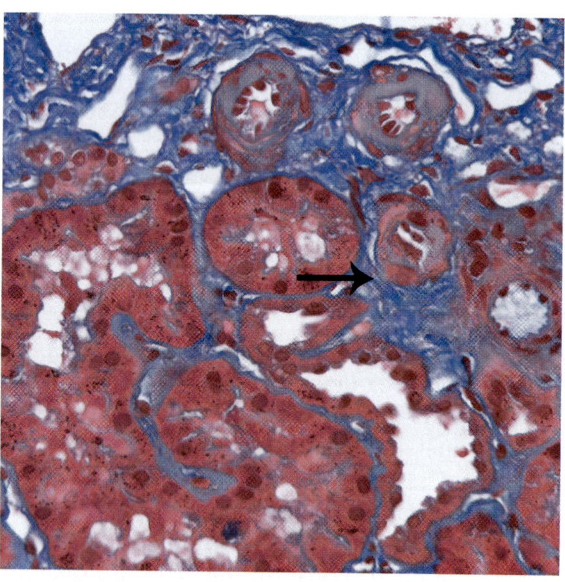

FIGURE 21.2. Chronic calcineurin inhibitor toxicity, peripheral nodules of hyaline are in an afferent arteriole, 2 years posttransplant (arrow; trichrome stain).

which are classically in a beaded pattern in the media. The usual hyaline deposits in hypertension or diabetes are subendothelial. The endothelial or smooth muscle cells may be vacuolated. Later biopsies show progressive scarring of arterioles, intimal fibrosis, and segmental glomerular obsolescence. Immunofluorescence of early lesions may show that the vessels have deposits of immunoglobulin M (IgM), C3, and fibrin. Electron microscopy shows apoptosis or necrosis of smooth muscle cells and replacement with hyaline material. Focal myocyte necrosis in the media of small arteries, in the absence of intimal changes, is regarded as a reliable indicator of CsA toxicity (3,4). The reversibility of the these lesions is debated.

Thrombotic Microangiopathy

Although more prevalent with higher doses of CsA in the 1980s, thrombotic microangiopathy (Fig. 21.3) still occurs under current regimens, even with careful attention to blood CsA levels. By 1994, the prevalence of CsA-associated thrombotic microangiopathy had decreased to 0.9%, accounting for 26% of the cases of thrombotic microangiopathy after renal transplantation (acute rejection, probably humoral, accounted for 53% and recurrent thrombotic microangiopathy 16%) (5). Patients typically present with acute renal failure, thrombocytopenia, microangiopathic hemolytic anemia, elevated lactic dehydrogenase, and hyperbilirubinemia. Despite these characteristic features, the clinical syndrome is not often recognized before biopsy. Those without systemic signs (thrombocytopenia, hemolysis) do considerably better (6).

The pathologic changes are the same as in thrombotic microangiopathy from other causes, although in the allograft the differential diagnosis with

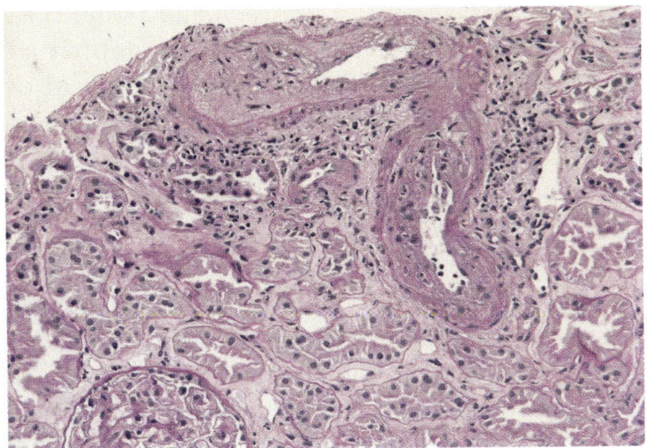

FIGURE 21.3. Acute calcineurin inhibitor toxicity due to tacrolimus, with a pattern of thrombotic microangiopathy that resembles endarteritis [periodic acid-Schiff (PAS) stain].

endarteritis can be challenging. Loose intimal thickening and trapped red cells are useful discriminators.

Differential Diagnosis

The criteria for the morphologic distinction of calcineurin inhibitor toxicity (CIT) and rejection have received much attention. Interstitial infiltrates are minimal in autologous kidneys with nephrotoxicity (5), but are common in early allografts, and have no differential value unless minimal. Patients with rejection typically have a diffuse, interstitial mononuclear cell infiltrate, whereas patients with CIT and those with stable function have only focal mononuclear cell infiltrates (7). Endarteritis is found rarely, if ever, in CIT (0–1%) and is the most discriminating feature between acute rejection and CIT (7,8). Among nine histologic features—(1) endarteritis, (2) interstitial edema, (3) distribution and (4) intensity of mononuclear cell interstitial infiltrate, (5) glomerulitis, (6) tubular ectasia, (7) tubular necrosis, (8) tubulitis, and (9) the ratio of mononuclear cells in the interstitium to those in peritubular capillaries—only the finding of endarteritis allowed the identification of rejection with any certainty (8). This agrees with my experience and that of others (4). Endothelial and medial smooth muscle cell vacuolization has been noted in CIT, best appreciated by electron microscopy. The frequency of vacuolization probably does not distinguish CIT from stable grafts (7).

Polyomavirus

Introduction/Clinical Setting

The BK polyoma virus virus was originally isolated from B.K., a Sudanese patient who had distal donor ureteral stenosis months after a living related transplant (9). BK virus is related to JC virus (which also inhabits the human urinary tract) and to simian kidney virus SV-40. These viruses are members of the papovavirus group, which includes the papilloma viruses. The BK virus commonly infects urothelium but rarely causes morbidity in immunocompetent individuals. However, in renal transplant recipients three lesions have been attributed to BK virus: hemorrhagic cystitis, ureteral stenosis, and acute interstitial nephritis (10,11). In a prospective study of 48 renal transplant recipients, active polyomavirus (BK or JC) infection was shown in 65%; 68% of these had intranuclear inclusions in urine cytology (12). Half of infections occurred within the first 3 months after transplantation, but some occurred 2 years or longer afterward. In 26% renal function became impaired at the time of the polyomavirus infection but no biopsy was done. A seropositive donor increased the rate of primary or reactivation infections with BK virus (13).

Pathologic Findings

Light Microscopy

The kidney shows interstitial nephritis, with mononuclear cells infiltrating the interstitium and tubules, often with a prominent component of plasma cells, which also may be occasionally found in tubules (Fig. 21.4) (14). Polyoma infection is initially suggested by the occurrence of markedly enlarged tubular epithelial cells with nuclear atypia and chromatin basophilia. The recognition of viral nuclear inclusions is the key step in diagnosis. The affected nuclei are usually enlarged and tend to be grouped in tubules; particularly collecting ducts in the cortex and outer medulla, and can often be spotted at low power. The mononuclear interstitial infiltrate is associated with the infected cells. Routine urine cytology readily reveals characteristic viral inclusions (decoy cells).

Immunohistochemistry

Polyomavirus large T antigen can be demonstrated in tubular epithelial cells, typically in clusters, and especially in collecting ducts (Fig. 21.5). Monoclonal antibodies are commercially available that react with BK specific determinants and with the large T antigen of several polyoma species. We have obtained good results with paraffin techniques. These techniques also work in urine cytology preparations.

Electron Microscopy

Electron microscopy reveals the characteristic intranuclear viral particles of 30–40-nm diameter in tubular epithelium (Fig. 21.6).

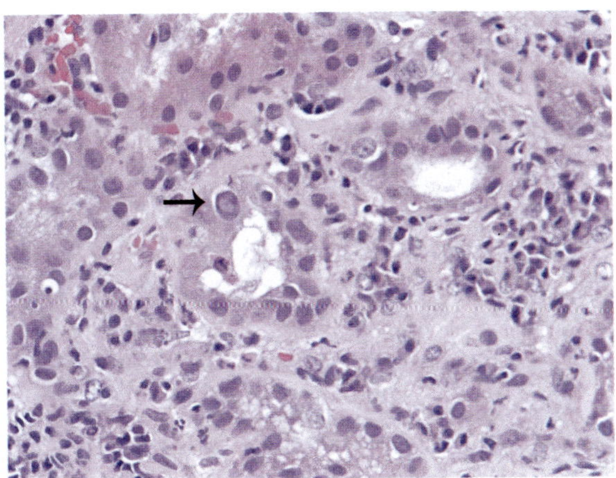

FIGURE 21.4. Polyomavirus interstitial nephritis. Plasma cells are abundant and nuclear inclusions are evident (arrow) (H&E stain).

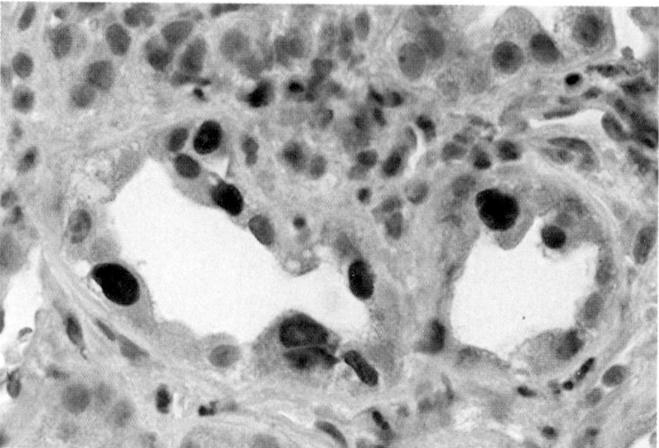

FIGURE 21.5. Polyomavirus interstitial nephritis. Viral antigens are demonstrated by immunoperoxidase stains in tubular epithelial nuclei using a monoclonal antibody to SV-40 large T antigen.

Pathogenesis

A promoting role for rejection appears likely, because polyomavirus interstitial nephritis is quite uncommon in recipients of heart, liver, or lung transplants. Alternatively, the allograft kidney may serve as a "sanctuary" for the virus, since T-cell killing of virally infected cells requires self–major

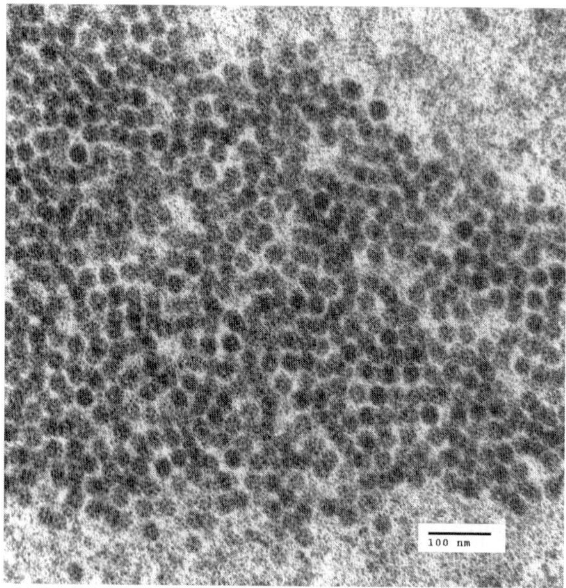

FIGURE 21.6. Polyomavirus interstitial nephritis. Electron microscopy reveals the 30- to 40-nm viral particles in tubular nuclei (bar = 100nm).

histocompatibility complex (MHC) antigens to be expressed on the target cells. Most recent cases have arisen in patients on tacrolimus or mycophenolate mofetil (MMF). Among centers using tacrolimus and MMF, the frequency of polyoma associated interstitial nephritis (AIN) is 3% to 5% (15–18). Recovery, without reduction of immunosuppression is not common (69% graft loss). With reduction of immunosuppression, graft survival is likely (>95%), but functional recovery is poor (38% have residual Cr >3.0 mg/dL) (15,17,19,20). Protocol biopsies and monitoring of blood/urine for virus should permit earlier treatment and improved outcome. The use of polymerase chain reaction (PCR) to detect viral DNA in the circulation has been reported to distinguish those with interstitial nephritis from noninvasive urothelial shedding of the virus (21). Antivirals, such as cidofovir, have had limited success.

Recurrent Renal Disease

The frequency and clinical significance of recurrence varies with the disease (14). The diseases that recur in >25% are dense deposit disease (90%), immunotactoid/fibrillary glomerulonephritis (GN) (67%), diabetes (>50%), IgA nephropathy (45%), Henoch-Schönlein purpura (33%), focal glomerular sclerosis (30%), idiopathic hemolytic uremic syndrome (27%), and type I membranoproliferative GN (27%). Lupus nephritis and anti-GBM disease recur infrequently (<5%). The diagnosis of recurrence requires accurate classification of the original disease and lesions that differ from chronic allograft glomerulopathy.

References

1. Mihatsch MJ, Thiel G, Ryffel B. Cyclosporine nephrotoxicity. Adv Nephrol Necker Hosp 17:303–320, 1988.
2. Mihatsch MJ, Thield G, Ryffel B. Morphologic diagnosis of cyclosporine nephrotoxicity. Semin Diagn Pathol 5:104–121, 1988.
3. Farnsworth A, Hall BM, Ng A, et al. Renal biopsy morphology in renal transplantation. Am J Surg Pathol 8:243–252, 1984.
4. Taube DH, Neild GH, Williams DG, et al. Differentiation between allograft rejection and cyclosporin nephrotoxicity in renal transplant recipients. Lancet 2:171–174, 1985.
5. Candinas D, Keusch G, Schlumpf R, Burger HR, Gmur J, Largiader F. Hemolytic-uremic syndrome following kidney transplantation: prognostic factors. Schweiz Med Wochenschr 124:1789–1799, 1994.
6. Schwimmer J, Nadasdy TA, Spitalnik PF, Kaplan KL, Zand MS. De novo thrombotic microangiopathy in renal transplant recipients: a comparison of hemolytic uremic syndrome with localized renal thrombotic microangiopathy. Am J Kidney Dis 41:471–479, 2003.

7. Neild GH, Taube DH, Hartley RB, et al. Morphological differentiation between rejection and cyclosporin nephrotoxicity in renal allografts. J Clin Pathol 39:152–159, 1986.
8. Sibley RK, Rynasiewicz J, Ferguson RM, et al. Morphology of cyclosporine nephrotoxicity and acute rejection in patients immunosuppressed with cyclosporine and prednisone. Surgery 94:225–234, 1983.
9. Gardner SD, Field AM, Coleman DV, Hulme B. New human papovavirus (B.K.) isolated from urine after renal transplantation. Lancet 1:1253–1257, 1971.
10. Nickeleit V, Hirsch HH, Binet IF, et al. Polyomavirus infection of renal allograft recipients: from latent infection to manifest disease. J Am Soc Nephrol 10:1080–1089, 1999.
11. Mylonakis E, Goes N, Rubin RH, Cosimi AB, Colvin RB, Fishman JA. BK virus in solid organ transplant recipients: an emerging syndrome. Transplantation 72:1587–1592, 2001.
12. Gardner SD, MacKenzie EF, Smith C, Porter AA. Prospective study of the human polyomaviruses BK and JC and cytomegalovirus in renal transplant recipients. J Clin Pathol 37:578–586, 1984.
13. Noss G. A serological investigation of BK virus and JC virus infections in recipients of renal allografts. J Infect Dis 158:176–181, 1988.
14. Colvin RB. Renal transplant pathology. In: Jennette JC, Olson JL, Schwartz MM, Silva FG, eds. Heptinstall's Pathology of the Kidney. Philadelphia: Lippincott-Raven, 1998:1409–1540.
15. Randhawa PS, Finkelstein S, Scantlebury V, et al. Human polyoma virus-associated interstitial nephritis in the allograft kidney. Transplantation 67:103–109, 1999.
16. Binet I, Nickeleit V, Hirsch HH, et al. Polyomavirus disease under new immunosuppressive drugs: a cause of renal graft dysfunction and graft loss. Transplantation 67:918–922, 1999.
17. Howell DN, Smith SR, Butterly DW, et al. Diagnosis and management of BK polyomavirus interstitial nephritis in renal transplant recipients. Transplantation 68:1279–1288, 1999.
18. Ramos E, Drachenberg CB, Papadimitriou JC, et al. Clinical course of polyoma virus nephropathy in 67 renal transplant patients. J Am Soc Nephrol 13:2145–2151, 2002.
19. Mathur VS, Olson JL, Darragh TM, Yen TS. Polyomavirus-induced interstitial nephritis in two renal transplant recipients: case reports and review of the literature. Am J Kidney Dis 29:754–758, 1997.
20. Drachenberg CB, Beskow CO, Cangro CB, et al. Human polyoma virus in renal allograft biopsies: morphological findings and correlation with urine cytology. Hum Pathol 30:970–977, 1999.
21. Nickeleit V, Klimkait T, Binet IF, et al. Testing for polyomavirus type BK DNA in plasma to identify renal-allograft recipients with viral nephropathy. N Engl J Med 342:1309–1315, 2000.

Index

I

R

S

Printed in the United States